PLAB 2 MASTER SERIES
VOLUME THREE
ADVANCED PRACTICE & MOCK OSCE
Practical Skills, Mock Stations and Final Sprint

AMaC · A. Mansour and Colleagues

PLAB 2 Master Series
Volume THREE: ADVANCED PRACTICE & MOCK OSCE
Practical Skills, Mock Stations and Final Sprint
AMaC (A. Mansour and Colleagues)

United Kingdom

Copyright

First published 2026.

ISBN (Paperback): 978-1-0667467-4-3

Published by AMaC (A. Mansour and Colleagues), United Kingdom.

CAUTION — Medical Disclaimer

The information contained in this book is intended solely for examination preparation purposes. It does not constitute clinical advice, medical guidance, or a substitute for professional medical judgement. The authors and publisher make no representations or warranties of any kind, express or implied, about the completeness, accuracy, or suitability of the information contained herein for clinical practice.

Clinical guidelines, drug doses, and protocols change. Readers must always consult current national guidelines, the British National Formulary (BNF), and senior clinical colleagues before applying any information in patient care.

The authors and publisher accept no liability for any loss, injury, or damage arising from the use of this material in any context other than PLAB 2 examination preparation.

Dedication

To those who sat the exam once and came back.
To those preparing to sit it for the first time with everything at stake.
To those who drive through the night to reach Manchester.

The finish line is learnable.

This volume shows you how to cross it.

Volume Three — ADVANCED PRACTICE & MOCK OSCE

AMaC — A. Mansour and Colleagues
United Kingdom, 2026

HOW TO USE VOLUME THREE

Volume Three builds on the communication and consultation skills developed in Volume One and the clinical medicine of Volume Two. It is designed to stand alone; the full series preface appears in Volume One.

This volume focuses on the practical and integrative skills tested in PLAB 2: systematic clinical examinations, bedside and ward procedures, ECG, ABG, chest X-ray and blood-test interpretation, prescribing safety, and the mock stations, timing maps and exam-day strategy that separate a pass from a fail. The emphasis is not on memorising guidelines, but on doing the right thing safely, in the right order, while verbalising clearly enough for the examiner to mark it.

Across procedures, examinations, data interpretation and the mock stations, the examiner is assessing the same core abilities:

✓ Recognise risk early

✓ Prioritise ABCDE and patient safety

✓ Escalate appropriately

✓ Communicate clearly and professionally

✓ Reassess after intervention

✓ Demonstrate safe NHS practice

Every chapter and station is structured around examiner expectations and focuses on the actions, verbalisation, and clinical reasoning that generate marks in the examination.

To maximise your score:

1. Read the chapter overview before studying the content.
2. Practise every examination and procedure aloud.
3. Learn the verbalisation scripts and Gold Closing Statements.
4. Review the Instant-Fail patterns in the data chapters (ECG, ABG, CXR, bloods).
5. Work the eighteen mock stations under timed conditions, then self-audit.
6. Use the final-sprint study plan in your last week.

Remember:

PLAB 2 is not primarily a test of medical knowledge. It is a test of whether you can recognise danger, manage uncertainty, communicate effectively, and keep patients safe.

The candidate who demonstrates safe clinical judgement will consistently outperform the candidate who simply knows the most facts.

AMaC Core Rule:

Recognise Early.
Act Safely.
Escalate Appropriately.
Reassess Frequently.
Think.
Speak.
Perform.

Table of Contents — Volume THREE

ADVANCED PRACTICE & MOCK OSCE

CHAPTER 57 · THE EXAMINATION FOUNDATION

VERBALISATION · SAFETY · CONSENT · CHAPERONE

Full Protocol Script · Every Station · All Specialties

CORE · 🔴 RED PATH · CAUTION — INSTANT FAIL RISK · EVERY STATION

Abbreviations used in this chapter: JVP Jugular Venous Pressure

DISTINCTION — Golden Triad of Fail — ANY ONE = very high risk of failing:

1. Silent examination — no verbalisation = no marks
2. No explicit consent before touching the patient
3. No chaperone offered for intimate examination

Also fail: Miss hand hygiene · Ignore patient pain or distress · Leave patient exposed unnecessarily

SAY — Examiner Rule: "Confidence and structure score more than rare sign detection. Slow hands, fast words."

Two-tier verbalisation: describe what you're DOING and what you're OBSERVING: "I'm gently pressing along the liver edge — still soft, no enlargement."

THINK — Core Mnemonics — Full Arsenal

Mnemonic	Use	Full Form
EXAMINE	Examination spine	Explicit consent · Xplain · Ask comfort · Minimal exposure · Involve chaperone · Never silent · End with summary
PREPARE	Patient-centred approach	Permission · Reason · Explain · Position · Ask comfort · Reassure · End
CONSENT	Consent process	Capacity · Open questions · No pressure · Sufficient info · Explicit verbal yes · Note · Time
CHAPERONE	Chaperone protocol	Check · Have trained · Always offer · Position · Explain role · Record · Offer same gender · Never if declined + uncomfortable · Escalate
COMFORT	Patient checks	Cover · Okay? · Modify · Feedback · Observe face · Reassure · Temperature · Hands warm

🔴 1. Before You Start — Universal Opening

Universal Opening Script:
"Hello, my name is [name], one of the doctors. Can I confirm your name and date of birth? With your permission, I'd like to examine your [area]. I'll explain everything as I go, and you can ask me to stop at any time. Before we begin, is there anything painful today?"
Privacy: "I'll close the curtains for your privacy." · Hand hygiene: "Before I start, I'll wash my hands." [Wash visibly] · Stethoscope: "I'll clean my stethoscope before using it."

CONSENT — Full Process:
C — Capacity (assume unless evidence otherwise) · O — Open questions: "Is it okay if I examine you?"
N — No pressure: "You can stop me at any time." · S — Sufficient info: "I need to examine your chest."
E — Explicit verbal yes (wait for "yes" — not just silence) · N — Note in records · T — Time: "Any questions before I start?"

2. Chaperone Protocol — Intimate Examinations

For INTIMATE EXAMS (breast, genitalia, rectum) — MUST offer chaperone:
"For this examination, it's routine to offer a chaperone — a trained member of staff who stays to support you. Would you like one present?"
Patient accepts → arrange before starting. Patient declines → are YOU comfortable alone? Yes → proceed + document "declined". No → escalate to senior.

C	Check	"Would you like a chaperone present?"
H	Have trained person	Ensure chaperone is appropriate and trained
A	Always offer	Breast, genital, rectal — every time, regardless of gender
P	Position	Chaperone visible throughout entire examination
E	Explain role	"They are here to support you."
R	Record	Document: offer, acceptance/decline, chaperone name
O	Offer same gender	Always offer regardless of examiner gender
N	Never examine if declined + uncomfortable	Escalate: "I'll ask a senior colleague to review with me."

3. During Examination — Verbalisation · Positioning · Comfort

Verbalisation Principle	Example
Say what you're doing	"I'm now palpating the abdomen gently."
Say what you see	"I can see the chest moving symmetrically."
Say what you find (positive)	"There is tenderness in the right iliac fossa."

Verbalisation Principle	Example
Say what's normal (NEGATIVE)	"There is no hepatomegaly · no ascites · no scars."
Explain as you go	"I'm now listening to your chest."
Compare both sides	"I'm comparing both sides systematically."

Pain-First Strategy: "Before I press, is there any area that is already painful?" · "I'll press gently first — tell me if you feel any pain."
If patient reports pain: "Thank you for telling me. I'll be gentler. Tell me immediately if it's too uncomfortable."
If patient winces: "I notice you're wincing — shall we pause? I'm sorry — can you show me exactly where it hurts?"
Comfort check every 30–45 seconds: "Are you okay? We're nearly finished."

Position	When	Script
Sitting upright	Chest / back	"Sit upright so I can examine properly."
45 degrees	Cardiovascular / JVP	"I'll adjust the bed to 45 degrees."
Lying flat	Abdominal	"Lie flat with arms by your side."
Any position	Always check	"Is that comfortable?"

When to STOP immediately: Patient expresses pain · withdraws consent · red flag finding · patient distressed · chaperone raises concern
"I'm noticing something important — I'll stop here and get a senior review immediately."

Intimate Exams (MAP) · Special Populations

MAP Protocol for Intimate Examinations:
M — Minimal exposure: expose only area needed, use gowns and towels
A — Always verbalise: "I'm now going to look at the area." — explain every action
P — Pause for comfort: watch face, check regularly — "Is this still okay? Tell me if you need me to stop."
After: "Thank you. I've finished. I'll help you cover up. Are you okay?" · Document: chaperone offered/accepted/declined, chaperone name.

Population	Approach	Script
Paediatric	Parent present · simple language	"I'll examine on your lap. We'll go slowly."
Cognitive impairment	Plain language · check understanding	"I'm going to touch your tummy. Is that okay?"
Language barrier	Professional interpreter	"I'll arrange an interpreter before we continue."

Population	Approach	Script
Hearing impairment	Face patient · speak clearly	"I'm facing you so you can see me."
Elderly	Support limbs · extra time	"I'll support your arm — tell me if it hurts."
Cultural sensitivity	Ask preferences	"Is there anything I should know before we begin?"

✓ 4. After Examination · Summary · Language Guide

Closing Script:
"Thank you — that's the end of the examination. I'll help you cover up. I'll clean my hands again." [Wash visibly]
Summary structure: (1) Positive findings (2) Negative findings (3) Interpretation (4) Next steps
"Breath sounds normal throughout, no added sounds. Expansion symmetrical. These findings suggest a normal respiratory examination."

✗ Never Say	✓ Say Instead
"This won't hurt."	"Tell me if it hurts."
"Relax."	"Take your time — let me know if uncomfortable."
"I'm just a student."	"I'm one of the doctors on the team."
"It's probably nothing."	"I'd like to check this with my senior."
"You don't mind, do you?"	"Would that be okay with you?"
"I'll just have a quick feel."	"I'm going to examine your abdomen."

Recovery Scripts:
Forgot consent: "I realise I didn't ask — is it okay if I examine you now?"
Forgot chaperone: "Before we continue, I must offer you a chaperone."
Caused pain: "I'm so sorry — I'll stop. Show me where it hurts."

Self-Audit Checklist — Every Station

Before + During ✓	After + Special ✓
✓ Explicit verbal consent before touching	✓ Negative findings verbalised
✓ Chaperone offered for intimate exam	✓ Both sides compared
✓ Hand hygiene before AND after	✓ Transitions smooth
✓ Stethoscope warmed / cleaned	✓ Red flags: stopped + escalated

Before + During ✓	**After + Special ✓**
✓ Every step verbalised	✓ Findings summarised (positive + negative)
✓ Patient comfort checked (≥2 times)	✓ Consent + chaperone documented
✓ Patient kept covered throughout	✓ Patient thanked + helped to cover
✓ Pain-first strategy used	✓ Recovery script if mistake made

Final Exam Mantra

EXAMINE: Explicit consent · Xplain · Ask comfort · Minimal exposure · Involve chaperone · Never silent · End with summary

CONSENT: Capacity · Open Qs · No pressure · Sufficient info · Explicit yes · Note · Time

CHAPERONE: Check · Have trained · Always offer · Position · Explain · Record · Offer same gender · Never if declined + uncomfortable · Escalate

NEVER: Examine in silence · Touch without consent · Intimate exam without chaperone offer · Miss hand hygiene · Ignore patient distress

Gold Closing:
"Introduce → confirm identity → explicit consent → offer chaperone → wash hands visibly → verbalise every step and every finding (positive AND negative) → pain-first strategy → check comfort every 30–45 sec → keep covered → transition smoothly → thank patient → summarise clearly."

Never examine in silence no marks without words	Explicit verbal consent wait for "yes"	Chaperone always offer breast, genitalia, rectum	Negative findings must be verbalised	Pain-first strategy ask before pressing
Slow hands fast words confidence = marks	Cover throughout dignity always	EXAMINE spine 7-step framework	Recovery scripts correct mistakes live	Both sides compare every system exam

TOP 5 EXAMINER Q&A · THE EXAMINATION FOUNDATION	
Q1. What must happen before you touch any patient?	Introduce yourself, confirm identity, explain the examination, gain consent, offer a chaperone, and wash your hands: every time.
Q2. When is a chaperone mandatory to offer?	Any intimate examination: breast, genital, rectal: and whenever the patient or you would feel safer with one; document the offer.
Q3. Why verbalise during examination?	Examiners can only mark what they see and hear: narrate findings and intentions throughout.
Q4. The patient declines part of the examination?	Respect it, explore concerns, explain the clinical reason, offer alternatives, and document the informed refusal.
Q5. How do you close every examination station?	Thank the patient, restore dignity and clothing, summarise findings aloud, and state your next steps and differentials.

TOP 5 EXAMINER Q&A · THE EXAMINATION FOUNDATION	
CURVEBALL	You forget a step midway through. Say so and correct it openly: "I should also have checked X: doing that now": insight scores; concealment fails.

CHAPTER 58 · CARDIOVASCULAR & RESPIRATORY EXAMINATION

Full Verbalisation Script · Systematic Sequence · Emergency Recognition · Differential Diagnosis

CORE · HIGH YIELD · COMMUNICATION HEAVY

Abbreviations used in this chapter: **COPD** Chronic Obstructive Pulmonary Disease · **HCM** Hypertrophic Cardiomyopathy · **JVP** Jugular Venous Pressure · **MCL** Mid-Clavicular Line · **RUQ** Right Upper Quadrant · **RV** Right Ventricle · **SVC** Superior Vena Cava · **VR** Vocal Resonance

DISTINCTION — Golden Triad of Fail:
1. Working in silence — verbalise EVERY step · 2. Missing peripheral examination before chest · 3. Forgetting JVP (CVS) or trachea/respiratory rate (Resp)
INSTANT FAILS: Skip peripherals · Forget JVP/trachea/RR · Auscultate through clothing · Percuss over scapula · No vocal resonance · No dynamic manoeuvres for murmur · Miss silent chest/tension pneumo without escalating

"Slow hands, fast words." — Two-tier verbalisation: describe what you're DOING and what you're OBSERVING.
Murmur found: TIME IT · LOCATE IT · RADIATION · MANOEUVRES · DIFFERENTIAL ·
Abnormal sounds: PERCUSSION · ADDED SOUNDS · VOCAL RESONANCE · DIFFERENTIAL

Emergency Recognition — Escalate Immediately

Pattern	Immediate Action + Script
Silent chest + respiratory distress	"Life-threatening asthma — no breath sounds in a breathless patient. High-flow O_2 + neb bronchodilators + senior NOW."
Tracheal deviation + hypotension + absent breath sounds	"Tension pneumothorax until proven otherwise. Senior NOW — prepare needle decompression."
Raised JVP + hypotension + muffled heart sounds	"Cardiac tamponade. Urgent echo + cardiology NOW."
Stridor	"Upper airway obstruction — immediate senior review NOW."
SpO_2 <92% + respiratory distress	"O_2 aiming 94–98%. Senior review."

PART 1: CARDIOVASCULAR EXAMINATION — PERFECT Mnemonic

P	Peripherals	Hands · radial pulse · BP · radio-femoral delay · collapsing pulse · peripheral pulses

E	Eyes & face	Conjunctival pallor · malar flush · corneal arcus · xanthelasma · central cyanosis
R	Region (JVP)	JVP at 45° · tracheal position · apex beat location
F	Feel	Apex beat character · heaves · thrills · carotid pulse character
E	Environment	Temperature · sacral oedema · ankle oedema
C	Chest auscultation	All 5 areas · both positions · bell vs diaphragm · carotid bruits
T	Tummy	Hepatomegaly · pulsatile liver · ascites

CVS Opening Script:
"Hello, I'm [name], one of the doctors. Can I confirm your name and DOB? I'd like to examine your heart. Is that OK? Chaperone available. I'll need you to remove your top and lie flat. I'll explain everything as I go. Any pain today? Before starting, I'll wash my hands and clean my stethoscope."

CVS Hand Sign	Script	Interpretation
Clubbing	"Nail angle loss."	Endocarditis, cyanotic heart disease
Splinter haemorrhages	"Dark lines under nails."	Endocarditis
Osler's nodes / Janeway	"Finger pulp nodules / palmar spots."	Endocarditis
Capillary refill	"5 sec pressure — <2 sec refill normal."	Peripheral perfusion

Radial Pulse: "Rate, rhythm, volume. Radio-radial delay → coarctation. Radio-femoral delay → coarctation."
Collapsing pulse: "Raise arm, feel for sharp tap at brachial pulse → aortic regurgitation."
Carotid: "Listen for bruits BEFORE palpating. One side at a time. Slow-rising=AS · Collapsing=AR · Bounding=CO_2 retention."

JVP — MUST DO (45°): Non-palpable · double waveform · changes with position/inspiration · occluded at base
"JVP elevated to [X cm] above sternal angle → right heart failure, fluid overload, or SVC obstruction."
Hepatojugular reflux: "Press RUQ for 10 sec — sustained JVP rise confirms right heart failure."

Apex Beat Character	Interpretation
Tapping	Mitral stenosis
Heaving/sustained	LV hypertrophy (pressure overload)
Thrusting/hyperdynamic	Volume overload (AR)

Apex Beat Character	Interpretation
Displaced	Cardiomegaly

Heaves vs Thrills: Heave = lifting sensation over LSE (RV hypertrophy). Thrill = palpable murmur (ball of hand over valve areas).
Left lateral roll: Brings out mid-diastolic murmur of mitral stenosis. Sit forward + expiration: brings out early diastolic of AR.

Auscultation Areas — "All Physicians Earn Too Much":
1. Aortic (2nd ICS, RSE) · 2. Pulmonary (2nd ICS, LSE) · 3. Erb's (3rd ICS, LSE) · 4. Tricuspid (4th/5th ICS, LSE) · 5. Mitral (5th ICS, MCL)
Bell lightly = low-pitched (MS). Diaphragm firmly = high-pitched (AR, rub). Listen for S1, S2, S3, S4, murmurs, rub.

Murmur	Timing	Best Heard	Radiation
Aortic stenosis	Ejection systolic	Aortic area	Carotids
Aortic regurgitation	Early diastolic	Left sternal edge	None
Mitral regurgitation	Pan-systolic	Apex	Axilla
Mitral stenosis	Mid-diastolic	Apex (bell)	None
TR	Pan-systolic	LLSB	Liver (louder on inspiration)
HCM	Ejection systolic	LLSB/apex	Valsalva louder, squat softer

Dynamic Manoeuvres: Left lateral=MS · Sit forward+expiration=AR · Squat=most louder (HCM softer) · Stand=HCM louder · Valsalva=HCM louder · Handgrip=MR/AR louder · Inspiration=right-sided murmurs

CVS Pattern	Likely Diagnosis
Displaced apex + pansystolic murmur radiating to axilla	Mitral regurgitation
Slow-rising carotid + ejection systolic to carotids	Aortic stenosis
Collapsing pulse + early diastolic at LSE	Aortic regurgitation
Raised JVP + oedema + hepatomegaly	Right heart failure
Tapping apex + mid-diastolic (bell, left lateral)	Mitral stenosis
Parasternal heave + loud P2	Pulmonary hypertension
Raised JVP + hypotension + muffled sounds	Cardiac tamponade — EMERGENCY

CVS Summary Template:
"Peripherally [no clubbing/splinters/Osler's]. JVP [normal/elevated]. Apex [normal/displaced/tapping]. Carotid [normal/slow-rising/collapsing]. Auscultation: [normal/S3/murmur consistent with...]. Oedema [absent/present]. Signs consistent with [diagnosis]. Differential: [list]. Investigations: ECG, echo, CXR, FBC, BNP."

PART 2: RESPIRATORY EXAMINATION — IPPA-C Mnemonic

I	Inspection	Hands · face · chest shape · breathing pattern · respiratory rate · trachea · lymph nodes
P	Palpation	Chest expansion · vocal fremitus · surgical emphysema
P	Percussion	All zones · comparing sides systematically · AVOID scapula
A	Auscultation	Breath sounds · added sounds · vocal resonance
C	Chest wall movement	Symmetry · accessory muscle use · intercostal recession

RESPIRATORY RATE — Count first, verbalise always: "The respiratory rate is [X] breaths per minute — [normal 12–20]."
CO_2 retention flap: "Ask patient to extend wrists — flapping tremor = type 2 respiratory failure."

TRACHEAL POSITION — MUST CHECK:
Away from affected side → tension pneumothorax (if distress) or large effusion · Towards affected side → collapse/fibrosis
"Tracheal deviation + distress + hypotension = tension pneumothorax until proven otherwise. EMERGENCY — senior + needle decompression."

Resp Sign	Interpretation	Priority
Clubbing	Lung cancer, bronchiectasis, fibrosis	High-yield
CO_2 flap	Type 2 respiratory failure	High-yield
Peripheral cyanosis	Poor oxygenation	High-yield
Barrel chest	COPD/emphysema	High-yield
Horner's (ptosis+miosis)	Pancoast tumour	Optional
Asymmetrical chest movement	Effusion, pneumothorax, collapse	High-yield

Percussion Zones — Systematic: Anterior (apices→lower) · Lateral (mid-axillary) · Posterior (supra-scapular → inter-scapular → infra-scapular, AVOID SCAPULA)
Resonant=normal · Hyperresonant=pneumothorax/COPD · Dull=consolidation/collapse · Stony dull=pleural effusion

Sound	Script	Interpretation	Emergency?
Fine crackles	"High-pitched, end-inspiratory, not cleared."	Fibrosis, early LVF	No
Coarse crackles	"Low-pitched, early, may clear with cough."	Pneumonia, bronchiectasis	No
Wheeze	"Musical, expiratory predominant."	Asthma, COPD	No
Stridor	"Inspiratory, loudest over trachea."	Upper airway obstruction	EMERGENCY
Bronchial breathing	"Harsh, hollow, expiration = inspiration."	Consolidation	No
Silent chest	"No breath sounds audible."	Life-threatening asthma/tension	EMERGENCY

Vocal Resonance — MUST DO: "Say '99' while I listen."
Increased (bronchophony/whispering pectoriloquy) = consolidation · Decreased = effusion/pneumothorax/collapse

Respiratory Pattern	Likely Diagnosis
Dull + bronchial breathing + increased VR	Consolidation
Stony dull + reduced breath sounds + reduced VR	Pleural effusion
Hyperresonant + absent breath sounds + reduced VR	Pneumothorax
Fine crackles + clubbing + normal percussion	Pulmonary fibrosis
Wheeze + hyperresonance + prolonged expiration	COPD/asthma
Coarse crackles + productive cough	Bronchiectasis/pneumonia
Silent chest + respiratory distress	Life-threatening asthma / tension pneumo — ESCALATE

Resp Summary Template:
"[RR X bpm] · [Trachea central/deviated] · [Expansion equal/reduced] · [Percussion resonant/dull/hyperresonant] · [Breath sounds vesicular/bronchial/reduced + added sounds] · [VR normal/increased/decreased] · [SpO_2 X%]. Signs consistent with [diagnosis]. Differential: [list]. CXR, ABG, FBC, CRP, sputum. If emergency — escalate immediately."

Differentiate Similar Findings

Finding A	Finding B	How to Differentiate
Dull percussion	Stony dull	Stony dull = effusion (absolute); dull = consolidation/collapse
Fine crackles	Coarse crackles	Fine = end-inspiratory, persists after cough; coarse = clears with cough
Wheeze	Stridor	Wheeze = expiratory, lower airway; stridor = inspiratory, over trachea
Heave	Thrill	Heave = lifting sensation (RV hypertrophy); thrill = palpable murmur
Displaced apex	Tapping apex	Displaced = cardiomegaly; tapping = palpable S1 = mitral stenosis

Examiner Checklist — Both Examinations

CVS ✓	Respiratory ✓
✓ Hand signs + capillary refill	✓ Respiratory rate counted + verbalised
✓ Radial pulse: rate, rhythm, volume	✓ CO_2 retention flap assessed
✓ Radio-femoral delay checked	✓ Tracheal position checked
✓ BP measured	✓ Chest expansion both sides
✓ Carotid: bruits before palpation	✓ Percussion systematic (not over scapula)
✓ JVP at 45° + hepatojugular reflux	✓ Added sounds identified + interpreted
✓ Apex located + characterised	✓ Vocal resonance assessed
✓ Heaves + thrills palpated	✓ Both sides compared at each zone
✓ All 5 areas auscultated	✓ Silent chest = emergency escalated
✓ Bell + diaphragm used	✓ Lymph nodes palpated
✓ Dynamic manoeuvres for murmur	✓ Oxygen saturation noted
✓ Sacral + ankle oedema	✓ Summary + differential + investigations

Final Exam Mantra

CVS — PERFECT: Peripherals · Eyes · Region (JVP) · Feel apex · Environment · Chest auscultation · Tummy
Resp — IPPA-C: Inspection · Palpation · Percussion · Auscultation · Chest wall movement
CVS never forget: JVP · left lateral roll for MS · sit forward for AR · carotid bruits before palpation
Resp never forget: Respiratory rate · trachea · systematic percussion · vocal resonance · silent chest = EMERGENCY
Emergencies: Silent chest=asthma · Deviation+hypotension=tension pneumo · Raised JVP+muffled+hypotension=tamponade · Stridor=senior NOW

Gold Closing:
"Systematic [CVS/Resp] examination completed. Findings: [summary]. Signs consistent with [diagnosis]. Differential: [2–3]. Investigations: [appropriate]. Emergency signs [absent/escalated immediately]."

PERFECT mnemonic CVS sequence	IPPA-C mnemonic Resp sequence	JVP at 45 degrees must verbalise	Trachea must check Resp non-negotiable	Count RR always basic vital sign
Vocal resonance after auscultation	Bell = MS diaphragm = AR	Stony dull = effusion not just dull	Silent chest EMERGENCY escalate	Murmur: TIME LOCATE radiation + manoeuvres

TOP 5 EXAMINER Q&A · CARDIOVASCULAR & RESPIRATORY EXAMINATION	
Q1. What must never be skipped at the start?	Peripheral signs: hands, pulse, blood pressure mention, face and eyes: the diagnosis often sits in the periphery.
Q2. Why is the JVP non-negotiable in CVS?	It is the bedside window on right heart filling: position at 45 degrees, look across the neck, and verbalise the height.
Q3. Where do you auscultate the heart?	All four valve areas plus the axilla for mitral radiation and carotids for aortic radiation, with the bell and diaphragm.
Q4. The respiratory examination's opening move?	Inspection counts: respiratory rate, work of breathing, and tracheal position before your stethoscope ever moves.
Q5. How do you present your findings?	A structured summary: peripheral signs, then central findings, then a differential and the investigations you would request.
CURVEBALL	You hear nothing abnormal. Normal is a finding: present a confident, complete negative examination: never invent murmurs to seem clever.

CHAPTER 59 · ABDOMINAL, THYROID & BREAST EXAMINATION

Full Verbalisation Script · ABDOMEN · PALPATE · THYROID+B · BREAST+CALM

CORE · HIGH YIELD · PATIENT-CENTRED · EVERY STATION

Abbreviations used in this chapter: DOB Date of Birth · LHC Left Hypochondrium · LIF Left Iliac Fossa · RHC Right Hypochondrium · RIF Right Iliac Fossa

THINK — First Question: "Have I introduced myself? Have I gained consent? Have I got a chaperone? Am I verbalising everything?"
Golden Rule: TALK CONTINUOUSLY — describe each step AND each finding (positive AND negative). Silence = no marks.
INSTANT FAIL: No consent · No chaperone (breast) · No hand hygiene · Silence · Negative findings not verbalised · Ignore patient discomfort · Miss escalation

Universal Opening + Closing:
Open: "Hello, I'm [name]. Name/DOB? I'd like to examine your [area]. I'll explain each step. Chaperone available. Expose just the area needed. Any pain? I'll wash my hands first."
Close: "Finished — thank you. Let me help you cover up. I'll wash my hands. To summarise: [positive findings] and [negative findings]. Next step: correlate with history."

PART 1: ABDOMINAL EXAMINATION — ABDOMEN + PALPATE

A	Appearance	Inspect: scars · distension · pulsations · masses · umbilicus
B	Bowel sounds	Auscultate BEFORE palpation · bruits over aorta/renals/iliacs
D	Dullness	Percuss all 9 regions · liver span · shifting dullness if suspected ascites
O	Organomegaly	Liver · spleen · kidneys — MUST check all three
M	Masses	Light then deep palpation all 9 regions
E	End: special tests	Only if indicated (Murphy's, Rovsing's, shifting dullness)
N	Negatives — verbalise all	Soft · non-tender · no masses · no organomegaly · normal bowel sounds

P	Position	"Lie flat, arms by sides, expose nipples to pubis."
A	Ask about pain	"Any tenderness? Tell me if anything hurts."
L	Light palpation	All 9 regions — no guarding, no rebound
P	Palpate deeply	All 9 regions — no deep masses
A	Assess organomegaly	Liver (RHC → medial) · Spleen (LHC → medial) · Kidneys (bimanual balloting)
T	Tenderness + special tests	Murphy's if cholecystitis · Rovsing's if appendicitis

E	Examine hernia orifices	Inguinal · femoral · umbilical — cough impulse

Auscultate BEFORE palpation (palpation can alter bowel sounds)
Red flags: Peritonism (guarding + rigidity) → STOP + urgent surgical review · Massive organomegaly → urgent imaging

Special Tests — Only If Indicated:
Murphy's: Press RHC, patient breathes in → pain/arrest = positive (cholecystitis)
Rovsing's: Press LIF → pain in RIF = positive (appendicitis)
Shifting dullness: Resonant → dull, patient rolls → dullness shifts = ascites

Abdominal Step	Master Negatives
Inspection	No scars, no distension, umbilicus central, no pulsations
Auscultation	Bowel sounds normal, no bruits
Light palpation	No tenderness, no masses in all 9 regions, no guarding
Deep palpation	No deep masses
Organomegaly	Liver/spleen not palpable, kidneys not ballotable
Hernia orifices	No cough impulse
Percussion	Normal resonance throughout, no shifting dullness
Summary	Abdomen soft, non-tender, no masses, no organomegaly

PART 2: THYROID EXAMINATION — THYROID+B

T	Turn (inspect from front)	No visible goitre · scars · masses · asymmetry
H	Hands on neck from behind	Palpate isthmus and lobes with neck slightly flexed
Y	You palpate isthmus	Isthmus normal, no nodules
R	Rotate to palpate lobes	Left lobe normal · right lobe normal · no nodules
O	Observe swallowing	"Swallow please — thyroid moves upward, no tenderness."
I	Isthmus re-check for tenderness	No tenderness
D	Deviation (tracheal position)	"Trachea central, no deviation."
L	Lymph nodes (cervical, systematic)	Pre/post-auricular, occipital, tonsillar, submandibular, anterior/posterior cervical, supraclavicular
B	Bruit (auscultate over lobes)	"No bruits heard."

RED FLAGS: Tracheal deviation → urgent imaging + specialist · Stridor → AIRWAY EMERGENCY — senior immediately

Special Tests — Only If Indicated: Pemberton's (arms raised → facial congestion = retrosternal goitre) · Lid lag (follow finger down)

Thyroid Step	Master Negatives
Inspection	No visible goitre, moves normally on swallowing
Palpation	Isthmus normal, lobes normal, no nodules, no tenderness
Swallowing test	Moves upward on swallowing
Lymph nodes	No cervical lymphadenopathy
Trachea	Central, no deviation
Auscultation	No bruits
Summary	Thyroid normal, no nodules, no nodes, trachea central

PART 3: BREAST EXAMINATION — BREAST+CALM

CAUTION — CRITICAL SAFETY — CHAPERONE REQUIRED:
Offer chaperone · Document offer + response · Chaperone present throughout · Re-confirm consent before touching
"For this examination, it's routine to offer a chaperone. Would you like one? Before I begin — is it still OK to proceed?"

B	Breasts exposed (inspection ×3)	Arms by sides → arms raised → hands on hips (pectoral tensed)
R	Raise arms	No tethering, no dimpling, symmetry maintained
E	Examine lying flat	Pillow under shoulder, hand behind head to flatten tissue
A	Axilla palpation	Support arm to relax pectoralis · all 4 walls: anterior, posterior, medial, lateral
S	Supraclavicular nodes	Palpate supraclavicular fossae bilaterally
T	Technique (quadrant/clock face)	Flat of fingers · all quadrants · central/areola · note nipple discharge
C	Comfort check	"Tell me if anything hurts" — check throughout
A	Axilla re-check	No axillary nodes
L	Lymph nodes (all)	No cervical, axillary, or supraclavicular nodes
M	Master negatives	Symmetrical · no skin changes · no lumps · no discharge · no nodes

RED FLAGS: Palpable lump → triple assessment (imaging + biopsy + specialist) · Axillary nodes → imaging + correlation

Breast Step	Master Negatives
Inspection (all 3 positions)	Symmetrical, no skin changes, no nipple changes, no visible masses
Inspection raised/hips	No tethering, no dimpling
Palpation (all quadrants)	No lumps, no tenderness in both breasts
Nipple	No discharge
Axilla (all 4 walls)	No axillary lymphadenopathy
Supraclavicular	No supraclavicular nodes
Summary	Breasts normal, no lumps, no lymphadenopathy

Critical Findings — Escalate Immediately

Finding	Action	Script
Peritonism (guarding + rigidity)	Urgent surgical review	"Signs of peritonism — stopping and escalating immediately."
Massive organomegaly	Urgent imaging	"Significant organomegaly — urgent imaging."
Tracheal deviation	Urgent imaging + specialist	"Tracheal deviation — urgent imaging and specialist review."
Stridor	Airway emergency	"Stridor — airway emergency. Senior NOW."
Breast lump	Triple assessment	"Palpable lump — triple assessment: imaging, biopsy, specialist."
Axillary nodes	Imaging + correlation	"Axillary nodes — correlate with breast, arrange imaging."

Examiner Checklist — All Three Examinations

Abdomen ✓	Thyroid ✓	Breast ✓
✓ Consent + hand hygiene	✓ Consent + hand hygiene	✓ Chaperone offered + documented
✓ Position flat	✓ Position sitting	✓ Consent re-confirmed before touching

Abdomen ✓	**Thyroid ✓**	**Breast ✓**
✓ Inspection all features	✓ Inspection + swallowing test	✓ Inspection ×3 positions
✓ Auscultate BEFORE palpation	✓ Palpate from behind	✓ Palpation (quadrant/clock)
✓ Light + deep (9 regions)	✓ Observe swallowing	✓ Axilla (all 4 walls)
✓ Liver + spleen + kidneys	✓ Cervical lymph nodes	✓ Supraclavicular nodes
✓ Hernia orifices	✓ Tracheal deviation	✓ Nipple area + discharge
✓ Percussion systematic	✓ Auscultate for bruits	✓ Master negatives verbalised
✓ Negatives verbalised	✓ Negatives verbalised	✓ Escalate if lump found

Final Exam Mantra

ABDOMEN: Appearance · Bowel sounds · Dullness · Organomegaly · Masses · End (special tests) · Negatives

PALPATE: Position · Ask · Light · Palpate deep · Assess organs · Tenderness · Examine hernia orifices

THYROID+B: Turn · Hands · You palpate · Rotate · Observe · Isthmus · Deviation · Lymph nodes · Bruit

BREAST+CALM: Breasts · Raise · Examine flat · Axilla · Supraclavicular · Technique · Comfort · Axilla · Lymph · Master negatives

Mini-summaries: Abdomen: "soft, non-tender, no masses, no organomegaly" · Thyroid: "normal, no nodules, no nodes, trachea central" · Breast: "normal, no lumps, no nodes"

Auscultate first before abdomen palpation	All 9 regions light then deep	Liver + spleen + kidneys all three organomegaly	Hernia orifices cough impulse	Thyroid from behind palpate + swallow test
Trachea always thyroid non-negotiable	Chaperone breast document always	Inspect ×3 arms down, raised, hips	Axilla 4 walls all walls systematically	Negatives always silence = no marks

TOP 5 EXAMINER Q&A · ABDOMINAL, THYROID & BREAST EXAMINATION	
Q1. Correct patient position for abdominal palpation?	Flat with arms by the sides, knees slightly relaxed, examining from the right, watching the face throughout.
Q2. What is the palpation sequence?	Light palpation of all nine regions away from pain first, then deep, then organs: liver, spleen, kidneys, then aorta.
Q3. Thyroid examination essentials?	Inspect, swallow test with water, palpate from behind, check lymph nodes, then assess thyroid status: hands, pulse, eyes, reflexes.

TOP 5 EXAMINER Q&A · ABDOMINAL, THYROID & BREAST EXAMINATION	
Q4. Non-negotiables in breast examination?	Chaperone offered and documented, full explanation and consent, systematic quadrants plus axillary tail and nodes.
Q5. How do you handle finding a mass?	Describe it systematically: site, size, shape, surface, consistency, mobility, tenderness: then state the referral pathway.
CURVEBALL	The patient winces before you touch the right iliac fossa. Examine that region last, watch the face not your hands, and verbalise the kindness: empathy is a marked behaviour.

CHAPTER 60 · NEUROLOGICAL & CRANIAL NERVE EXAMINATION

Full Verbalisation Script · OSCE-Adapted Systematic Examination

CORE · SYSTEM EXAM · HIGH YIELD · Stroke · Elderly · A&E

Abbreviations used in this chapter: **CN** Cranial Nerve · **EOM** Extraocular Movements · **ICP** Intracranial Pressure · **LMN** Lower Motor Neurone · **LP** Lumbar Puncture · **MRC** Medical Research Council scale · **SAH** Subarachnoid Haemorrhage · **UMN** Upper Motor Neurone

DISTINCTION — Golden Triad of Fail:

1. Missing focal weakness without escalation · 2. Not comparing reflexes side-to-side · 3. Incomplete cranial nerve examination

INSTANT FAIL: Silence · No MRC scale · No left-right comparison · No coordination · Miss pupil examination · Focal deficit not escalated

SAY — Examiner Rule: "Confidence and structure score more than rare sign detection. Compare left AND right. Grade everything."

OSCE-adapted screen: Prioritise limbs over detailed cranial nerves unless indicated. If time limited: UL → LL → Gait → CN screen.

THINK — UMN vs LMN — Must Know

Feature	UMN	LMN
Tone	↑ Spastic (clasp-knife)	↓ Flaccid
Reflexes	↑ Brisk (3+/4+)	↓ / Absent
Plantar	↑ Extensor (Babinski +)	↓ Flexor (normal)
Wasting	Late / none	Early and prominent
Fasciculations	Absent	Present
Clonus	May be present	Absent

PARTS 1–3: LIMB EXAMINATION — Tone · Power (MRC) · Reflexes · Coordination · Sensation

MRC Power Scale: 0=No movement · 1=Flicker · 2=Gravity eliminated · 3=Against gravity · 4=Against resistance · 5=Normal

Reflexes: 0=Absent · 1=Diminished · 2=Normal · 3=Brisk · 4=Clonus · ALWAYS compare left vs right

Upper Limb	Lower Limb	Negatives Script
Tone: passive movement of wrist/elbow	Tone: roll leg, ankle clonus	"Tone normal both sides. No clonus."

Upper Limb	Lower Limb	Negatives Script
Power: shoulder, elbow, wrist, grip, fingers	Power: hip, knee, ankle, great toe	"Power 5/5 throughout."
Reflexes: biceps (C5-6), triceps (C7), supinator	Reflexes: knee (L3-4), ankle (S1), plantar	"Reflexes 2+ equal. Plantars flexor."
Coordination: finger-nose, dysdiadochokinesia	Coordination: heel-shin	"Coordination intact."
Sensation: light touch, pinprick, vibration, proprioception (DIP)	Sensation: light touch, pinprick, vibration (malleolus), proprioception (great toe)	"Sensation normal all modalities, symmetrical."

Pronator drift — HIGH YIELD for stroke: "Arms out, palms up, eyes closed — hold 10 sec." Downward drift + pronation = contralateral UMN.
Extensor plantar (Babinski): Stroke lateral sole → great toe extends = UMN lesion.
Clonus: If reflexes 3+, check with sudden ankle dorsiflexion. Sustained beats = UMN.

Gait + Romberg:
Normal gait: "Walk to end of room and turn." Look for symmetry, arm swing, balance.
Tandem gait: "Heel-to-toe in a straight line." Cerebellar ataxia fails.
Romberg: "Feet together, eyes open then closed." Falls eyes closed only = sensory ataxia (posterior column).

PART 4: CRANIAL NERVE EXAMINATION — CN II–XII

CN II + III (pupils): Must examine. Papilloedema = raised ICP = escalate immediately.
30-Second Screen: "CN II–XII intact — pupils equal, eye movements full, face symmetrical, hearing intact, palate central, shoulder shrug strong, tongue central."

Cranial Nerve	Test	Normal Script
CN I Olfactory	Not routinely tested unless history indicates	
CN II Optic	Visual acuity (Snellen) · fields (confrontation) · pupils (direct + consensual) · fundoscopy if indicated	"Acuity 6/6. Fields full. Pupils equal and reactive."
CN III/IV/VI	"Follow my finger — don't move your head." H-pattern. Note nystagmus, diplopia.	"EOM full. No nystagmus. No diplopia."
CN V Trigeminal	Motor: clench teeth. Sensory: V1/V2/V3 (forehead, cheek, chin).	"Motor normal. Sensation intact all 3 divisions."
CN VII Facial	Upper: raise eyebrows, screw eyes shut. Lower: show teeth, puff cheeks.	"Facial movements symmetrical. Eye closure strong."

Cranial Nerve	Test	Normal Script
CN VIII Vestibulocochlear	Whisper a number in each ear (covered).	"Hearing grossly intact bilaterally."
CN IX/X	"Open wide, say Ah." Palate elevation. Sip of water. Voice clear.	"Palate central. Swallow normal. Voice clear."
CN XI Accessory	Shoulder shrug + head rotation against resistance.	"Shoulder shrug and head rotation strong."
CN XII Hypoglossal	"Stick out your tongue." Note deviation, wasting, fasciculations.	"Tongue central. No wasting. No fasciculations."

CN VII — UMN vs LMN: UMN = forehead sparing (bilateral cortical input to upper face). LMN = complete facial weakness including forehead.
CN XII: Tongue deviates TOWARDS side of LMN lesion.

DANISH — Cerebellar Signs

D — Dysdiadochokinesia · A — Ataxia · N — Nystagmus · I — Intention tremor · S — Speech (scanning) · H — Hypotonia

Localisation — Pattern Recognition

Finding Pattern	Localisation
Distal symmetrical weakness + areflexia	Peripheral neuropathy
Proximal weakness + normal reflexes	Myopathy
UMN signs + aphasia	Dominant hemisphere (stroke)
UMN signs + sensory level on trunk	Spinal cord
LMN one limb only	Nerve root / peripheral nerve
Ataxia + nystagmus + intention tremor	Cerebellar
Crossed signs (face one side, body other)	Brainstem
Inconsistent findings	Functional neurological disorder

Localisation Template:
"This patient has [right-sided UMN signs] with [increased tone, brisk reflexes, extensor plantar]. This localises to the [left corticospinal tract]. Most likely: [acute stroke]. I would correlate with history and arrange [investigations]."

RED FLAGS — HOT-BACK-TRAUMA — Escalate Immediately

On identifying any focal deficit — STOP further testing and ESCALATE IMMEDIATELY: "I've identified [focal weakness/papilloedema/sensory level]. I will stop and escalate immediately to my senior."

H	Head injury + neuro signs	Urgent CT head
O	Onset sudden (stroke)	Stroke pathway + check glucose immediately
T	Trauma + neuro deficit	Immobilise + trauma CT
B	Back pain + leg weakness	Urgent MRI spine
A	Acute visual loss	Urgent ophthalmology
C	Cauda equina (saddle + retention + bilateral legs)	MRI spine + surgical review — SURGICAL EMERGENCY
K	Kernig's sign + fever + neck stiffness	IV antibiotics immediately + LP
T	Thunderclap headache (SAH)	CT head + LP if CT negative

Examiner Checklist — Self-Audit

Limb Examination ✓	**CN + Safety ✓**
✓ Explicit consent + hand hygiene	✓ CN II: acuity + fields + pupils
✓ General inspection (speech, posture, tremor)	✓ CN III/IV/VI: EOM + nystagmus
✓ UL tone + power (MRC) + reflexes	✓ CN VII: forehead (UMN vs LMN distinction)
✓ Pronator drift checked	✓ CN IX/X: palate + swallow
✓ LL tone + clonus + power + plantars	✓ CN XII: tongue central + no fasciculations
✓ Left vs right compared throughout	✓ DANISH cerebellar signs assessed
✓ Coordination: finger-nose + heel-shin	✓ HOT-BACK-TRAUMA red flags screened
✓ Sensation all 4 modalities	✓ Focal deficit → escalated immediately
✓ Gait + Romberg	✓ Localisation attempted
✓ Negatives verbalised throughout	✓ Summary + differential + investigations

Final Exam Mantra

UMN: Tone↑ · Reflexes↑ · Plantar↑ (Babinski) · No wasting · Clonus
LMN: Tone↓ · Reflexes↓ · Flexor plantar · Early wasting · Fasciculations
MRC 0–5: No movement → flicker → gravity eliminated → against gravity → against resistance → normal
DANISH: Dysdiadochokinesia · Ataxia · Nystagmus · Intention tremor · Speech · Hypotonia
HOT-BACK-TRAUMA: Head · Onset sudden · Trauma · Back+legs · Acute visual · Cauda equina · Kernig · Thunderclap

Gold Closing:
"Systematic neuro examination: UL/LL tone, power (MRC), reflexes (left vs right), plantars, coordination, sensation, gait, Romberg, CN II–XII. Localisation: [finding]. Most likely: [diagnosis]. Investigations: [next steps]. Focal deficit [absent/escalated]."

MRC scale 0-5 always grade power	Reflexes 0-4 always compare L vs R	Plantar reflex extensor = UMN	Pronator drift high-yield stroke sign	DANISH cerebellar all 6 signs
CN II + III pupils non-negotiable	CN VII forehead UMN vs LMN key	HOT-BACK-TRAUMA escalate immediately	Cauda equina surgical emergency	Localise always synthesise findings

THINK — GCS Component Reference — Always State E/V/M Separately

CAUTION — NEVER give GCS as total alone. Always state all three components.

Eye (E): E4=Spontaneous — E3=To voice — E2=To pain — E1=None
Verbal (V): V5=Oriented — V4=Confused — V3=Words — V2=Sounds — V1=None
Motor (M): M6=Obeys — M5=Localises — M4=Withdraws — M3=Flexion — M2=Extension — M1=None

Example: GCS 10 = E3, V3, M4 — state each. GCS ≤8: airway protection required — involve anaesthetics immediately.

TOP 5 EXAMINER Q&A · NEUROLOGICAL & CRANIAL NERVE EXAMINATION	
Q1. How do you keep a full neuro exam inside OSCE time?	Structure beats completeness: tone, power, reflexes, sensation, coordination per limb: verbalising as you go: offer to complete what time cuts.
Q2. Power grading you must verbalise?	MRC 0–5: state the grade per movement: "hip flexion 4 out of 5 on the left".
Q3. The cranial nerve shortcuts that lose marks?	Skipping visual fields, fundoscopy mention, or gag-reflex consideration: name them even when offering to complete later.
Q4. Upper vs lower motor neuron signs?	UMN: increased tone, brisk reflexes, upgoing plantars. LMN: wasting, fasciculations, reduced tone and reflexes.
Q5. How do you finish?	Summarise the pattern: where is the lesion, what is the lesion: then the investigations that would confirm it.
CURVEBALL	Cerebellar signs appear in a "routine" limb exam. Pivot aloud: "this changes my differential: I would now formally assess coordination, gait and speech".

CHAPTER 61 · MUSCULOSKELETAL & GALS EXAMINATION

GALS · LOOK–FEEL–MOVE–FUNCTION · NHE (Shoulder) · LMV (Knee) · TTF (Hip)

VERY HIGH YIELD · CAUTION — COMMUNICATION HEAVY · HIGH STAKES

Abbreviations used in this chapter: **ACL** Anterior Cruciate Ligament · **MCL** Medial Collateral Ligament · **MCP** Metacarpophalangeal joint · **MTP** Metatarsophalangeal joint · **TMJ** Temporomandibular Joint

DISTINCTION — Golden Fail Triad:

1. No gait observation · 2. No 3 screening questions · 3. Miss hot swollen joint

INSTANT FAILS: Skip Look–Feel–Move–Function · Work in silence · No functional assessment · Don't compare sides · Miss joint above and below · Cauda equina not escalated

SAY — Core Rule: "Interpret every finding aloud. If you don't observe gait and ask the 3 screening questions, I fail you."

ALWAYS: Examine joint ABOVE and BELOW (referred pathology). Compare BOTH SIDES.

GALS SCREEN — Gait · Arms · Legs · Spine

3 Screening Questions — ASK FIRST, EVERY TIME:

"Any pain or stiffness in your muscles, joints, or back?" · "Any difficulty dressing yourself?" · "Any problems going up or down stairs?"

G	Gait	Walk/turn/heel-toe. Inspect footwear for uneven wear. Antalgic=painful joint. Trendelenburg=hip abductor weakness.
A	Arms	Inspection · upper limb movements · grip · pinch · MCP squeeze. Tenderness=inflammatory arthritis (RA).
L	Legs	Inspection · squat (hip/knee/ankle) · patellar tap + bulge sign · hip log roll · MTP squeeze. Tenderness=early RA.
S	Spine	Inspect front/back/side (scoliosis, kyphosis, lordosis) · touch toes · lateral flexion · thoracic rotation · cervical · TMJ.

GALS Summary Script:

"GALS complete. Gait normal. Arms: full movement, MCP not tender. Legs: full squat, MTP not tender. Spine: normal curves, full flexion. TMJ normal. No red flags. Patient performs daily activities normally."

LOOK–FEEL–MOVE–FUNCTION — Universal Joint Exam

L	Look	Swelling · deformity · wasting · skin changes · scars — all angles
F	Feel	Temperature · tenderness · effusion · crepitus — warn before palpating

M	Move	Active THEN passive · range · pain · instability — compare both sides
F	Function	Squat · stairs · grip · reach · dress — "Can you perform daily activities?"

SHOULDER — NHE: Neer · Hawkins · Empty Can

Step	Action	Script
Look	Deltoid wasting · AC joint swelling · scars	"Inspecting for deltoid wasting, AC joint swelling."
Feel	AC joint · supraspinatus · biceps tendon	"Any tenderness here? Feeling for warmth."
Move	Active: abduction, forward flex, ER, behind back. Then passive.	"Raise arm to side. Forward. Now I move it."
Function	Overhead reach · behind back · cross-body adduction	"Reach above head. Touch back of neck."
N — Neer	IR + forward flexion	"Painful arc 60–120° = subacromial impingement."
H — Hawkins	90° abduction + IR	"Hawkins + Neer positive = impingement confirmed."
E — Empty Can	Scapular plane, thumb down, resist downward force	"Weakness = supraspinatus tear."

Shoulder Summary: "No wasting. Full range. Neer/Hawkins negative, empty can strong = normal. If impingement: X-ray + physio."

KNEE — LMV: Lachman · McMurray · Valgus Stress

Step	Action	Script
Look	Effusion · quad wasting · valgus/varus · scars	"Effusion, quad wasting, alignment."
Feel	Temperature · joint line · patellar tap · bulge sign	"Warm? Joint line tender? Patellar tap + bulge."
Move	Active + passive: flexion, extension, crepitus	"Bend and straighten. Feeling for crepitus."
Function	Squat · step-up · sit-to-stand	"Can you squat? Step up and down?"
L — Lachman	Tibia drawn forward at 30° flexion	"Most sensitive for ACL rupture."
M — McMurray	Flex, extend, rotate — click or pain	"Positive = meniscal tear."

Step	Action	Script
V — Valgus Stress	Valgus force at 30° flexion	"Laxity = MCL injury."

Knee Summary: "No swelling. Full flexion/extension. No effusion. Lachman firm, McMurray negative, stable valgus = normal. If mechanical: X-ray + physio."

HIP — TTF: Thomas · Trendelenburg · FABER

Step	Action	Script
Look	Gait (antalgic/Trendelenburg) · standing + lying	"Antalgic=painful. Trendelenburg=hip abductor weakness."
Feel	Greater trochanter · groin tenderness	"Over greater trochanter and groin."
Move	Flexion · extension · abduction · adduction · log roll (IR)	"Knee to chest. Log roll — reduced IR = earliest OA sign."
Function	Walk · stairs · sit-to-stand	"Stairs? Sit/stand without help?"
T — Thomas	Flex one hip maximally — other leg rises	"Thomas positive = fixed flexion deformity."
T — Trendelenburg	Single-leg stand — pelvis drops on unsupported side	"Positive = hip abductor weakness."
F — FABER	Flexion–Abduction–External Rotation	"Groin pain = hip. Buttock pain = SI joint."

Hip Summary: "Normal gait. Full range, IR preserved. Thomas/Trendelenburg/FABER negative. If OA: AP + lateral hip X-ray."

RED FLAGS — HOT-BACK-TRAUMA · Inflammatory vs Mechanical

HOT-BACK-TRAUMA — Escalate Immediately:

HOT: Hot swollen joint + fever → Septic arthritis until proven otherwise — orthopaedics + bloods + aspiration NOW. DO NOT inject local anaesthetic into the joint before aspirating — it dilutes culture and may be unsafe.

BACK: Back pain + bladder/bowel dysfunction + saddle anaesthesia → Cauda equina — emergency MRI + neurosurgical referral TODAY

TRAUMA: Trauma + inability to weight bear → Fracture — X-ray immediately

Feature	Inflammatory	Mechanical
Pain timing	Morning stiffness >30 min, improves with activity	Worse with activity, better with rest
Night pain	Common — wakes patient	Uncommon

Feature	Inflammatory	Mechanical
Swelling	Soft tissue / effusion	Bony swelling
Systemic	Fever, fatigue, weight loss	None
Examples	RA, PsA, AS, gout, septic arthritis	OA, trauma, meniscal tear

Finding Pattern	5-Second Diagnosis
Symmetrical small joints + morning stiffness >30 min	Rheumatoid arthritis
DIP joints + Heberden/Bouchard nodes	Osteoarthritis
Acute monoarthritis + fever + hot joint	SEPTIC ARTHRITIS — emergency
Knee locking + giving way	Meniscal tear — MRI
Knee swelling within 2h of trauma	ACL rupture — urgent MRI
Groin pain + reduced internal rotation	Hip OA — AP + lateral X-ray
Shoulder painful arc 60–120°	Subacromial impingement
Back pain + bladder/bowel + saddle anaesthesia	Cauda equina — emergency MRI NOW
First MTP acute swelling + redness	Gout — uric acid + aspiration

Examiner Checklist

GALS + Joint Exam ✓	RED FLAGS + Interpretation ✓
✓ 3 screening questions asked	✓ HOT joint + fever = septic — escalated
✓ Gait observed (antalgic/Trendelenburg)	✓ Cauda equina symptoms checked
✓ Footwear inspected	✓ Trauma + weight bearing asked
✓ MCP squeeze (arms)	✓ Inflammatory vs mechanical differentiated
✓ Squat + MTP squeeze (legs)	✓ Findings verbalised continuously
✓ Spine + TMJ examined	✓ Both sides compared
✓ LOOK–FEEL–MOVE–FUNCTION in order	✓ Joint above + below examined
✓ NHE (Neer, Hawkins, Empty can)	✓ Function assessed
✓ LMV (Lachman, McMurray, Valgus)	✓ Investigations stated
✓ TTF (Thomas, Trendelenburg, FABER)	✓ Safety-net provided

Final Exam Mantra

GALS: 3 questions → Gait → Arms (MCP) → Legs (MTP/squat) → Spine (TMJ)

Joint exam: LOOK–FEEL–MOVE–FUNCTION always in order · NHE (Shoulder) · LMV (Knee) · TTF (Hip)

HOT = septic (escalate NOW) · BACK = cauda equina (emergency MRI) · TRAUMA = X-ray immediately

High-yield: MCP tender=RA · Reduced hip IR=OA · Painful arc 60–120°=impingement · Lachman=ACL · McMurray=meniscus

Gold Closing:

"GALS: [normal/abnormal]. Gait [normal/antalgic/Trendelenburg]. Arms MCP [not tender]. Legs MTP [not tender], full squat. Spine full range. No red flags. Patient performs daily activities normally. Investigations: [X-ray/MRI/bloods/physio/referral]."

3 screening questions before any GALS	Gait first always observe before touching	MCP squeeze inflammatory = tender	MTP squeeze early RA sign	NHE shoulder Neer Hawkins Empty can
LMV knee Lachman McMurray Valgus	TTF hip Thomas Trendelenburg FABER	HOT joint = septic escalate NOW	Cauda equina emergency MRI today	Joint above + below always examine both

TOP 5 EXAMINER Q&A · MUSCULOSKELETAL & GALS EXAMINATION	
Q1. What is the GALS screen?	Gait, Arms, Legs, Spine: a rapid screen with three questions: pain or stiffness, dressing, stairs.
Q2. The regional exam structure?	Look, Feel, Move, Function: inspection, palpation, active then passive movement, then what the joint must do in life.
Q3. What must you never miss in a hot swollen joint?	Septic arthritis: say it, and state that aspiration before antibiotics is the rule.
Q4. Why compare both sides?	Asymmetry is the diagnosis half the time: always expose and compare the contralateral joint.
Q5. Special tests: how do you use them?	Name the test, the structure it stresses, and the finding: a named negative scores more than an unnamed positive.
CURVEBALL	The patient cannot fully undress due to pain. Adapt and verbalise: examine what is accessible, support the limb, and state what full assessment would add: pragmatism with dignity scores.

CHAPTER 62 · MENTAL STATE EXAMINATION — FULL VERBALISATION SCRIPT

ASEPTIC Framework · RISK Screen · AMT-10 · Insight · Biopsychosocial Formulation

CORE · HIGH YIELD · PATIENT-CENTRED · Psychiatry · GP · Acute

Abbreviations used in this chapter: AMT-10 Abbreviated Mental Test (10-point) · **MSE** Mental State Examination

THINK — First Question: "Is this patient safe? Are they at risk of harm to self or others?" — RISK screen BEFORE MSE.

INSTANT FAIL: No RISK assessment · Miss command hallucinations · Miss thought possession · Forget insight · Forget cognition (elderly/confusion) · Confront delusions · No summary with formulation

SAY — Golden Minute Opening: "Hello, I'm Dr [Name]. Before we start, I ask everyone: have you had thoughts of harming yourself or ending your life? [If yes: Thank you for telling me — important so I can keep you safe.] We can take breaks. Is that OK?"

RISK Screen — Pre-MSE Safety (Do FIRST)

R — Risk to self: "Have you had thoughts of harming yourself or ending your life?"
I — Intent / plan / means: "Do you have a plan? What stops you? Do you have access to [method]?"
S — Self-neglect: "Are you eating, drinking, looking after yourself? Do you feel safe at home?"
K — Known others at risk: "Have you had thoughts of harming anyone else?"

Risk Level	Indicators	Action
LOW	Passive thoughts · no plan · strong supports	Safety plan + routine follow-up
MODERATE	Ideation + some intent · limited supports	Crisis team · 48–72h review
HIGH	Plan + intent + means · recent attempt	Escalate urgently · consider admission

THINK — ASEPTIC — Full MSE Framework

A	Appearance & Behaviour	Observe throughout. Dress · grooming · eye contact · posture · rapport · psychomotor changes
S	Speech	Rate · rhythm · volume · tone · form (logical/tangential/circumstantial/flight of ideas/thought blocking)

E	Emotion/Mood	Subjective ("how have you been feeling?") + Objective (euthymic/depressed/elevated) · affect range/reactivity/congruence
P	Perception	Hallucinations (all modalities) · command hallucinations MUST ask · illusions · depersonalisation
T	Thought	Form (logical/tangential) + Content (delusions · obsessions · thought possession: insertion/withdrawal/broadcasting)
I	Insight	1. Aware of illness? · 2. Attributes symptoms? · 3. Willing to accept treatment?
C	Cognition	AMT-10 if: elderly · confusion · falls · delirium screen · memory complaint

SAY — Perception · Thought · Insight — Key Questions

Perception — Always Ask:
"Have you heard voices when no one was around?" · "What do they say?" · "Do the voices EVER tell you to do things?" — COMMAND HALLUCINATIONS
"Have you seen things others can't see?" · Illusions · depersonalisation · derealisation

Thought Content — Must Ask All:
"People watching you or out to get you?" (paranoid) · "Special powers or mission?" (grandiosity)
"Thoughts INSERTED into your mind? Taken OUT? BROADCAST so others can hear them?" — THOUGHT POSSESSION
"Thoughts that keep coming back despite trying to stop them?" (obsessions)
Cultural sensitivity: "I'm not here to challenge your beliefs — I want to understand your experiences."

Thought Form Types:
Logical=normal · Circumstantial=delayed but returns · Tangential=moves off, doesn't return · Flight of ideas=rapid + pressured · Thought blocking=sudden stop
Insight — 3 components: (1) Aware of illness? · (2) Attributes symptoms to illness? · (3) Willing to accept treatment?

THINK — Cognition — AMT-10

Q	Question	Score
1	Age	/1
2	Time (nearest hour)	/1
3	Address for recall: 42 West Street (ask now, test at end)	(recall later)
4	Year	/1
5	Name of hospital / location	/1

Q	Question	Score
6	Recognition of two persons	/1
7	Date of birth	/1
8	Widely known historical fact	/1
9	Count backwards 20–1	/1
10	Recall address (42 West Street)	/1
TOTAL	≤10 = normal · ≤7 = cognitive impairment · ≤3 = significant impairment	/10

Delirium Triad — Escalate Immediately: Acute onset + fluctuating consciousness + visual hallucinations → urgent medical review

Pattern Recognition · Formulation · Escalation

Presentation Pattern	Likely Diagnosis
Pressured speech + flight of ideas	Mania
Flat affect + poverty of speech + negative symptoms	Schizophrenia
Acute onset + fluctuating attention + visual hallucinations	DELIRIUM — urgent medical review
Low mood + psychomotor retardation + anhedonia	Depression
Obsessions + compulsions + insight retained	OCD
Progressive memory loss + disorientation	Dementia

Biopsychosocial Formulation:
"This appears to be a [predisposed] patient, precipitated by [trigger], maintained by [perpetuating factors], protected by [strengths]."
Escalation: Low risk: safety plan + GP follow-up · Moderate: crisis team + 48h review · High: escalate urgently to psychiatry · consider admission
Capacity: If refuses + high risk → MCA test: Understand · Retain · Weigh · Communicate

Examiner Checklist

ASEPTIC Domains ✓	Risk + Formulation ✓
✓ RISK screen done first	✓ Command hallucinations asked
✓ Appearance + behaviour described	✓ Thought possession asked (insertion/withdrawal/broadcasting)
✓ Speech: rate, rhythm, form	✓ Cultural context considered

ASEPTIC Domains ✓	Risk + Formulation ✓
✓ Mood: subjective + objective	✓ AMT-10 if elderly/confusion/falls
✓ Affect: range, reactivity, congruence	✓ Insight: 3 components assessed
✓ Perception: all modalities	✓ Risk stratified: low/moderate/high
✓ Thought form + content	✓ Protective factors stated
✓ Delusions explored	✓ Biopsychosocial formulation given
✓ Capacity if high risk + refusal	✓ Summary + escalation + safety-net

Final Exam Mantra

RISK first · ASEPTIC framework · OBSERVE → EXPLORE → TEST → FORMULATE
NEVER miss: command hallucinations · thought possession · insight · cognition in at-risk · summary with formulation
AMT-10: elderly, confusion, falls, delirium screen · Capacity: MCA 4 tests if high risk + refusal
Cultural context BEFORE labelling beliefs as pathological · Never confront delusions

Gold Closing:
"Appearance [describe]. Speech [rate/form]. Mood subjectively [words] · objectively [euthymic/depressed/elevated] · affect [full/restricted], [congruent/incongruent]. Thought form [logical/tangential]. Content [delusions/possession]. Perception [no hallucinations / auditory, 2nd/3rd person, no commands]. AMT-10 [X/10]. Insight [full/partial/none]. Risk [low/moderate/high] · protective factors [X]. Formulation: predisposed [X], precipitated [Y], maintained [Z]. Plan: [safety plan / refer / escalate urgently]."

RISK screen first before any MSE domain	Command hallucinations must always ask	Thought possession insertion withdrawal broadcast	Insight 3 components awareness attribution Rx	AMT-10 elderly confusion falls
Subjective vs objective both mood required	Affect range + congruence not just flat/elevated	Cultural context before labelling beliefs	Delirium triad acute+fluctuating +visual	Formulation 4Ps predispose precipitate perp protect

TOP 5 EXAMINER Q&A · MENTAL STATE EXAMINATION	
Q1. The MSE domains in order?	Appearance and behaviour, speech, mood and affect, thought form and content, perception, cognition, insight: plus risk.
Q2. Mood vs affect?	Mood is the patient's sustained subjective state; affect is what you observe moment to moment: report both.
Q3. How do you screen thought content safely?	Ask directly about hopelessness, suicidal thoughts, plans and intent, and thoughts of harming others: every MSE includes risk.

TOP 5 EXAMINER Q&A · MENTAL STATE EXAMINATION	
Q4. Assessing insight in one move?	"What do you yourself think is happening?": their explanation tells you insight, beliefs, and engagement at once.
Q5. Cognition when time is short?	Orientation to time, place and person at minimum: offer formal cognitive testing as the next step.
CURVEBALL	The patient is guarded and gives one-word answers. Your observations ARE the examination: describe appearance, rapport, eye contact and psychomotor state richly: silence is data.

CHAPTER 63 · CANNULATION, VENEPUNCTURE & ABG SAMPLING

Safe Procedures · ANTT · Aseptic Technique · CANNULA · VEIN · ABG SAFE

CORE · PROCEDURAL SKILL · HIGH YIELD

Abbreviations used in this chapter: ABG Arterial Blood Gas · ANTT Aseptic Non-Touch Technique · AV Arteriovenous · EDTA Ethylenediaminetetraacetic Acid (blood tube additive) · PVD Peripheral Vascular Disease

DISTINCTION — Golden Principle: Safety > Sterility > Success
INSTANT FAIL: No consent · Breach ANTT · Tourniquet >2 min · Skip Allen's test (ABG) · Recap needle · 2 failed attempts without escalating · Miss/ignore complications

SAY — Universal Verbalisation: "Washing hands. Maintaining ANTT throughout. Sharp scratch coming. Tourniquet released. Flashback confirmed. Flushing. Needle to sharps bin immediately."

Cannula Size Guide

Size	Colour	Typical Use
24G	Yellow	Fragile veins / paediatrics
22G	Blue	Routine adults
20G	Pink	Most fluids / medications
18G	Green	Blood transfusion / trauma
16G	Grey	Major resuscitation

CANNULATION — CANNULA Mnemonic

C	Consent	"Explicit verbal consent confirmed. Sharp scratch. Explain each step."
A	Aseptic	Hand hygiene · gloves · clean tray · maintain ANTT throughout
N	Needle / Site	Select distal vein first · bevel up 15–20° · antecubital fossa preferred
N	Numb if needed	Local anaesthetic if patient anxious
U	Use tourniquet	<2 minutes — RELEASE before needle withdrawal
L	Line insertion	Flashback seen → advance cannula → flush 0.9% saline to confirm patency
A	Aftercare	Dressing · secure · safety-net · document · needle to sharps bin immediately

Extravasation: Swelling around cannula → STOP infusion immediately, remove cannula, apply pressure

VENEPUNCTURE — VEIN Mnemonic

V	Vein selection	Antecubital fossa preferred · distal veins first
E	Equipment ready	Needle · tubes · holder · tourniquet · cotton wool
I	Insert at 15–20°	Bevel up · flashback confirms entry · attach tubes in order
N	Needle withdrawal	Release tourniquet FIRST · apply pressure 1–2 min · label tubes at bedside

Tube order: Culture → Coagulation → Serum → EDTA/Other · Always label at bedside before leaving patient

ABG SAMPLING — ABG SAFE Mnemonic

Allen's Test — MANDATORY before every radial ABG: Compress both radial + ulnar arteries → hand blanches → release ulnar → hand flushes pink <5 sec = PASS. If fails = use alternative site.

A	Allen's test	Mandatory radial check before every attempt. Failed = use alternative site.
B	Brachial/Radial	Palpate strongest pulse · radial preferred
G	Gas collection	1–2 mL · NO air bubbles — expel air to avoid false PaO_2
S	Syringe capped + mixed	Cap immediately · mix to prevent clotting
A	Apply pressure	5 min normal · 10 min if anticoagulated
F	Flush if delayed	On ice if analysis delayed >10 minutes
E	Escalate if complication	Bleeding · haematoma · nerve injury → STOP and escalate

Contraindications to radial ABG: Failed Allen's test · AV fistula · severe PVD · local infection · previous radial artery harvest

CAUTION — Complications — Recognise + Act

Complication	Recognition	Action
Haematoma	Swelling / bruising at site	Firm pressure + elevate limb
Arterial bleed	Pulsatile bright red blood	Sustained pressure ≥10 min · escalate immediately
Nerve injury	Sharp / electric pain during procedure	STOP immediately · escalate to senior

Complication	Recognition	Action
Vasovagal	Pallor, sweating, dizziness	Lie flat, legs up, reassure, monitor
Anaphylaxis	Rash, wheeze, hypotension	Call help · IM adrenaline · oxygen · IV access
Extravasation	Swelling / coolness around cannula	Stop infusion · remove cannula · pressure

Aftercare · Documentation · Sharps

Pressure times: Cannula removal: 1–2 min · ABG: 5 min (normal) · 10 min (anticoagulated)

Sharps: NEVER recap. Dispose directly into sharps bin at point of use.

Documentation: "Indication · site · cannula size · number of attempts · complications · flush success · patient tolerance."

Safety-net: "If you feel numbness, increasing pain, swelling, or bleeding — inform staff immediately."

2 failed attempts: Escalate to senior. Do NOT attempt a third time alone.

Examiner Checklist

Procedure ✓	Safety + Aftercare ✓
✓ Explicit consent obtained	✓ Tourniquet released before withdrawal
✓ Hand hygiene + ANTT maintained	✓ Sharps disposed at point of use (no recap)
✓ Correct cannula size selected	✓ Pressure applied (correct time)
✓ Distal vein first	✓ Documentation stated
✓ Allen's test (ABG)	✓ Safety-net given
✓ Air expelled (ABG)	✓ Complications recognised + acted on
✓ Tube order correct (venepuncture)	✓ Escalated after 2 failed attempts
✓ Flashback confirmed	✓ Patient comfort checked

Final Exam Mantra

PREPARE → PERFORM → AFTERCARE · Safety > Sterility > Success

CANNULA: Consent · Aseptic · Needle/site · Numb · Use tourniquet (<2 min) · Line · Aftercare

VEIN: Vein selection · Equipment · Insert 15–20° · Needle withdrawal

ABG SAFE: Allen's (mandatory) · Gas (no air) · Pressure 5/10 min · Ice if delayed · Escalate

NEVER: Recap needle · Tourniquet >2 min · Skip Allen's · 3 attempts alone

Safety first consent + ANTT always	Allen's test mandatory before ABG	Tourniquet <2 min release before withdrawal	No recap ever direct to sharps bin	Flashback = confirm before advancing

Air = false PaO2 expel from ABG syringe	Pressure 5/10 min ABG normal/anticoag	2 attempts = escalate not three alone	Tube order Culture-Coag-Serum-EDTA	Label at bedside never before taking blood

TOP 5 EXAMINER Q&A · CANNULATION, VENEPUNCTURE & ABG SAMPLING	
Q1. What does ANTT actually require at the bench?	Key parts stay sterile and untouched: clean the site 30 seconds and let it dry: never repalpate after cleaning.
Q2. Sharps rules that fail candidates?	Take the sharps bin to the patient, dispose immediately yourself, never resheath, never hand a sharp to anyone.
Q3. Failed first cannulation attempt: what now?	Acknowledge, apologise, reassess: new device, new site, maximum two attempts, then call for senior or specialist help.
Q4. Before an ABG, what must you do?	Explain that it is painful, consent, perform/mention the modified Allen test, and state local anaesthetic consideration.
Q5. After any blood draw?	Pressure on the site, label at the bedside, document, and tell the patient what happens with the results.
CURVEBALL	Blood spills onto the trolley mid-procedure. Verbalise safety: glove change, clean per spillage protocol, fresh key parts: composure under contamination is the test.

CHAPTER 64 · CATHETERISATION — MALE & FEMALE

PREPARE · CLEAN-GO · CLEAN-SEE · CUFI · R-F-R · CARE · DRAIN · D-T-C-B-B-U-T

CORE · HIGH YIELD · PROCEDURE HEAVY

Abbreviations used in this chapter: **CAP** Community-Acquired Pneumonia

DISTINCTION — Golden Triad of Fail:
1. Inflate balloon before urine return · 2. Break sterility and continue · 3. No chaperone offered (female)

INSTANT FAILS: Balloon without urine (urethral trauma) · Force against resistance · Vaginal insertion without marker · No R-F-R after 3 min · No chaperone · No CARE instructions

SAY — Golden Rules: "PREPARE first. Urine before balloon — always. Vaginal insertion: leave as marker, use new catheter. R-F-R by 3 minutes. Never force."
STOP Rule: S=Sharp pain · T=Trickles blood · O=Obstruction · P=Patient distressed → Stop immediately.

MALE CATHETERISATION — CLEAN-GO

C	Clean	Urethral meatus · circular motion · centre outward
L	Lube	10–20 mL lidocaine gel · wait 3–5 minutes
E	Erect	Hold penis at 90°
A	Advance	Gently until urine flows — NEVER FORCE
N	No force	Stop if resistance · patient deep breaths · reassess
G	Go (CUFI)	Advance 5–6 cm further once urine flows → inflate balloon (CUFI)
O	Out	Connect bag · secure · REDUCE FORESKIN (prevent paraphimosis) · document

Foreskin: ALWAYS reduce foreskin to natural position after male catheterisation. Failure = paraphimosis.

FEMALE CATHETERISATION — CLEAN-SEE

C	Clean	Labia and urethra · front to back
L	Locate (CLUE)	Identify urethral meatus: between clitoris (anterior) and vaginal orifice (posterior) · torch if needed
E	Entry	Aim slightly upward · advance gently

A	Advance	Until urine flows + advance 2–3 cm further
N	No vagina	If entered: LEAVE IN PLACE as marker · use NEW catheter above it
S	Secure	Connect bag · secure to thigh · BBNK (Below Bladder · No Kinks)
E	End	Document · give CARE aftercare

Vaginal insertion recovery: LEAVE catheter in vagina as anatomical marker. Insert NEW catheter into urethra ABOVE it. Remove vaginal catheter ONLY after new one is confirmed in bladder.

CUFI Balloon Safety · R-F-R Troubleshooting

CUFI — Balloon Safety (Both Male + Female):
C — Check: urine is flowing freely · U — Urine confirmed in bladder · F — Fill balloon slowly · I — Inflate while watching patient for pain
Standard balloon: 10 mL. NEVER inflate without confirmed urine return.

R-F-R — No Urine by 3 Minutes: START IMMEDIATELY and verbalise:
R — Reposition: rotate/withdraw slightly · check for kinks
F — Flush: 10 mL sterile water — NEVER force
R — Replace: remove + use new catheter if still no urine
Script: "No urine yet — starting R-F-R: reposition, flush with 10 mL sterile water, replace if needed."

Aftercare · Documentation · Removal

CARE Instructions — Give Every Time:
C — Clean daily (soap + water) · A — Assess bag (empty at ⅔ full · below bladder · no kinks · BBNK) · R — Review need (remove ASAP) · E — Empty safely
Hydration: 1.5–2 L daily unless fluid restricted.
Seek help if: No urine 4–6h · pain · fever · blood · catheter falls out · confusion

D-T-C-B-B-U-T Documentation:
Date · Time · Catheter size + type · Balloon volume · Batch number · Urine (appearance + volume) · Tolerance (comfort + complications)

DRAIN — Catheter Removal:
Deflate (confirm water volume) · Remove gently · Assess spontaneous void · Instruct (report if no void 6–8h) · Note PVR
Post-Void Residual: <100 mL = normal · 100–200 mL = monitor · >200 mL = retention → ISC + urology referral
Suprapubic catheter: ASSESS ONLY. NEVER insert or manipulate — surgical procedure.

CAUTION — Complications · Contraindications · CAUTI Prevention

Complication	Recognition	Action
Haematoma	Swelling / bruising at site	Firm pressure + elevate
Arterial bleed	Pulsatile bright red blood	Sustained pressure ≥10 min · escalate
Nerve injury	Sharp/electric pain during procedure	STOP · escalate
Paraphimosis	Foreskin swelling after male cath	Reduce foreskin ALWAYS post-procedure
CAUTI	Fever · cloudy urine · dysuria	Sterile technique · closed system · review daily
False passage	Difficulty advancing + pain	Stop · never force · senior review

> Contraindications — B-P-S-R-C: Blood at meatus · Pelvic fracture · Stricture · Refusal · Chaperone absent (female) → STOP

Examiner Checklist

Procedure ✓	**Safety + Aftercare ✓**
✓ PREPARE + verbal consent	✓ Urine confirmed BEFORE balloon (CUFI)
✓ Chaperone offered (female)	✓ CUFI: 10 mL · patient observed
✓ Allergies: latex + iodine	✓ Foreskin reduced (male)
✓ Hand hygiene + sterile field	✓ BBNK confirmed
✓ Contraindications checked	✓ R-F-R if no urine by 3 min
✓ Meatus identified (CLUE female)	✓ CARE instructions given
✓ Vaginal marker: left as guide	✓ Seek-help criteria stated
✓ Never forced against resistance	✓ D-T-C-B-B-U-T documented
✓ STOP rule applied if resistance	✓ Catheter need: daily review stated

Final Exam Mantra

PREPARE → CAP (consent+chaperone+allergies) → hand wash → sterile field
CLEAN-GO (male): Clean · Lube · Erect · Advance · No force · Go (CUFI) · Out + FORESKIN
CLEAN-SEE (female): Clean · Locate · Entry · Advance · No vagina · Secure · End
CUFI: urine flowing → 10 mL balloon → watch patient · R-F-R if no urine by 3 min
CARE aftercare · D-T-C-B-B-U-T documentation · BBNK bag position · STOP rule always

Gold Closing:

"Catheter inserted using sterile technique. [X] mL urine drained. CUFI: 10 mL balloon after confirmed urine. BBNK confirmed. Foreskin reduced (male). D-T-C-B-B-U-T documented. CARE instructions given: daily clean, bag below bladder, 1.5-2 L fluid, remove ASAP. Return if no urine 4-6h, pain, fever, or blood."

Urine before balloon always CUFI rule	10 mL balloon standard volume	Never force STOP rule	Foreskin always prevent paraphimosis	Vaginal marker leave + new catheter
R-F-R at 3 min reposition flush replace	BBNK bag below bladder no kinks	Chaperone female non-negotiable	Suprapubic assess only never insert	D-T-C-B-B-U-T full documentation

TOP 5 EXAMINER Q&A · CATHETERISATION	
Q1. The consent conversation must include?	Why it is needed, what it involves, discomfort, risks (infection, trauma, bleeding), alternatives, and a chaperone offered and documented.
Q2. The one mistake that causes urethral trauma?	Inflating the balloon before urine flows: never balloon without urine: advance fully, see urine, then inflate.
Q3. Male catheter will not pass: what next?	Stop forcing: more anaesthetic gel, adjust angle, smaller or coudé consideration: then urology: force is the fail.
Q4. Aseptic essentials at the field?	Sterile field, clean from front to back/centre outward, one hand stays sterile, anaesthetic gel given time to work.
Q5. After insertion, what completes the station?	Connect drainage, secure, record residual volume, restore dignity, document size/balloon/residual, and plan review for removal.
CURVEBALL	Frank haematuria appears in the bag. Stop and reassess aloud: traumatic vs pre-existing, monitor, escalate to urology: do not silently carry on.

CHAPTER 65 · SUTURING & WOUND CARE

SAFE TIE · WOUND · DIRTY · LA TIP · TIE · TIMING · INFECT · CARE · DOC · STOP

CORE · HIGH YIELD · PATIENT-CENTRED

Abbreviations used in this chapter: **BNF** British National Formulary

DISTINCTION — Golden Triad of Fail:
1. Break sterility and continue · 2. Close a DIRTY wound primarily · 3. No chaperone offered (intimate areas)

INSTANT FAILS: No tetanus check · Inject without aspirating · No sensation test · Tie too tight (tissue blanching) · No edge eversion · No TIMING or INFECT aftercare

SAY — Golden Rule: "SAFE TIE first. WOUND before closure. DIRTY = never close primarily. Evert edges, not too tight. Aftercare saves patients."

STOP Rule: Sharp pain · Trickles blood · Obstruction · Patient distressed → STOP and reassess immediately.

1. Pre-Procedure — SAFE TIE · WOUND · DIRTY · Tetanus

S	Sterile field	Sterile pack · gloves · drape
A	Allergy check	"Any allergies to latex, lidocaine, or iodine?"
F	First aid / haemostasis	Control bleeding before starting
E	Examine wound	Depth · contamination · neurovascular status
T	Time since injury	<6h limbs/trunk · <12h face (primary closure window)
I	Irrigate	Thoroughly with saline until visibly clean
E	Explore	Foreign bodies · tendon · nerve · vessel · bone

DIRTY — Do NOT Close Primarily (any ONE = leave open):
Delayed (>6h limbs, >12h face) · Infected/contaminated · Risk to tendon/nerve/bone · Trauma (animal/human bite) · Young/immunocompromised

Tetanus: Fully vaccinated + clean = no action. Fully vaccinated + tetanus-prone = booster if >10yr. Unknown/incomplete = booster + consider immunoglobulin.

Tetanus-prone: Deep · contaminated · puncture · bites · burns

Exploration: Test distal sensation + full ROM (tendon) + capillary refill + pulses. "Exploring — no foreign bodies. Tendon and nerve intact distally."

2. Local Anaesthesia — LA TIP · Irrigation

LA TIP:
L — Lidocaine 1% (check BNF max dose) · A — Aspirate BEFORE injecting · T — Test sensation after 2–5 min · I — Inject slowly · P — Perpendicular, 3–5 mm from edge
Adrenaline CAUTION: Avoid in digits · nose · penis · ears (end-arteries)

Irrigation: Saline (first choice) · Clean tap water (acceptable alternative) · Povidone-iodine (dilute, contaminated only) · Hydrogen peroxide: NOT recommended (damages tissue)
Script: "You'll feel a sharp scratch and burn. Aspirating before injecting. Testing sensation before starting."

3. Closure — TIE Technique · Suture Selection · Dressing

T	Take suture	Perpendicular · 3–5 mm from edge · same depth both sides
I	Instrument loop	Wrap suture around needle driver TWICE (first throw)
E	End with square knot	Second throw opposite direction · third throw same direction (1-2-1)

3 Non-Negotiable Points:
1. Evert edges (lift slightly while tying — prevents depressed scar)
2. Not too tight — tissue must NOT blanch (ischaemia = poor healing)
3. Evenly spaced (width of suture apart — even tension)

Site	Suture type	Removal
Face	Fine sutures (cosmesis)	5 days
Scalp	Stronger	7 days
Trunk	Standard	10 days
Limbs	Stronger	10–14 days
Joints	Vertical mattress (tension)	10–14 days

Alternatives to sutures: Tissue glue (small, low-tension, face, children) · Steri-strips (superficial adjunct) · Staples (scalp, limbs — remove 7–10 days)
Bite wounds: Irrigate copiously · leave open · consider co-amoxiclav · ID team for PEP (Hep B, tetanus, HIV) · assess rabies risk

4. Aftercare — INFECT · CARE · DOC

INFECT — Warning Signs (must explain to patient):
Inflammation (redness/swelling) · Nasty discharge (pus) · Fever >38°C · Erythema spreading beyond edges · Crepitus · Tenderness increasing
Crepitus = gas in tissues = EMERGENCY → A&E IMMEDIATELY

CARE Aftercare:
C — Check wound daily (redness, swelling, discharge) · A — Advise removal: "Remove in [X] days at your GP"
R — Reassure healing: "Scar fades over months — protect from sun 6–12 months, massage with moisturiser" · E — Escalate if INFECT signs develop

DOC Documentation: Date · Wound description · Tetanus status · Sutures used · Aftercare plan · Follow-up arranged

Examiner Checklist

Pre-Procedure + Wound ✓	**Closure + Aftercare ✓**
✓ SAFE TIE checklist followed	✓ Irrigation with saline
✓ Consent + chaperone offered	✓ Exploration (foreign body, tendon, nerve)
✓ Allergy: latex, lidocaine, iodine	✓ LA TIP: aspiration + sensation test
✓ Tetanus status checked	✓ Adrenaline caution known
✓ Neurovascular assessment	✓ TIE: perpendicular, 1-2-1 knot
✓ WOUND mnemonic applied	✓ Edges everted
✓ DIRTY criteria checked	✓ Not too tight, no blanching
✓ Sterile field maintained	✓ TIMING by site given
✓ Bite wound: ID + PEP if applicable	✓ INFECT signs explained (crepitus=A&E)
✓ STOP rule if resistance	✓ DOC documentation completed

Final Exam Mantra

SAFE TIE: Sterile · Allergy · First aid · Examine · Time · Irrigate · Explore
WOUND + DIRTY before closure · DIRTY = never close primarily
LA TIP: aspirate + test sensation · No adrenaline in digits/nose/penis/ears
TIE: perpendicular + evert + not too tight + 1-2-1 knot
TIMING: Face 5d · Scalp 7d · Trunk 10d · Limbs 10–14d · Joints 10–14d
INFECT: crepitus = A&E emergency · CARE aftercare · DOC · STOP rule

Gold Closing:
"SAFE TIE followed. Wound assessed: WOUND + DIRTY criteria — suitable for primary closure. Tetanus, allergies, neurovascular checked. Irrigated. Explored: no FB, tendon/nerve intact. LA TIP: aspirated + sensation confirmed. TIE: perpendicular, evert, not too tight, 1-2-1. Dressing applied. TIMING: [site] — [X] days. INFECT warning given. CARE: check daily, advise removal, sun protection. DOC completed."

SAFE TIE first universal checklist	WOUND + DIRTY before any closure	Aspirate before inject LA non-negotiable	Test sensation 2-5 min after LA	Evert edges prevents scar depression
Not too tight no tissue blanching	TIMING by site face 5 to joints 14	Crepitus = A&E INFECT emergency	Bite = leave open ID + PEP assess	STOP rule pain/blood/obstruction

TOP 5 EXAMINER Q&A · SUTURING & WOUND CARE	
Q1. Before any suture touches skin?	Assess the wound: mechanism, depth, structures, contamination: check tetanus status, and consider neurovascular and tendon injury.
Q2. Local anaesthetic safety in one line?	State the agent, maximum dose (lidocaine 3 mg/kg plain), aspirate before injecting, and warn of the sting.
Q3. Which wounds must you NOT close?	Bites, heavily contaminated or devitalised wounds, and deep punctures: irrigate, consider delayed closure, antibiotics per protocol.
Q4. The suturing technique markers?	Instrument handling, needle at 90 degrees, square knots, even spacing and eversion: narrate each step.
Q5. What completes wound care?	Irrigation volume verbalised, dressing, tetanus and antibiotic decisions stated, safety-netting for infection, and removal timing.
CURVEBALL	Movement of the finger is weak after a palm laceration. Stop: suspected tendon injury is not for ED closure: examine, document, splint and refer to hand surgery.

CHAPTER 66 · AIRWAY ADJUNCTS, OXYGEN THERAPY & CHEST DRAINS

OPA · NPA · BMV (SEAL) · Oxygen (O_2 SAFE) · WISE · SWAB · LAT · SUCTION

CORE · 2026 RED PATH · Oxygen Errors INSTANT FAIL

Abbreviations used in this chapter: **BMV** Bag-Mask Ventilation · **COPD** Chronic Obstructive Pulmonary Disease · **MCL** Mid-Clavicular Line · **NIV** Non-Invasive Ventilation · **NPA** Nasopharyngeal Airway · **OPA** Oropharyngeal Airway

DISTINCTION — Golden Triad of Fail:

1. High-flow O_2 to stable COPD without Venturi mask → CO_2 retention → respiratory arrest
2. OPA in conscious patient (gag reflex intact) → vomiting → aspiration
3. Clamp chest drain without senior instruction → tension pneumothorax

INSTANT FAILS: No SpO_2 target documented · NPA in skull fracture · One-person BMV · No suction ready · No reassessment after O_2 · Drain not below chest · Ignoring continuous bubbling

SAY — Golden Rule: "Oxygen is a drug — prescribe with a target. Venturi for stable COPD. Two-person BMV always. Never clamp without senior instruction. Verbalise every step. Escalate early."

AIRWAY ADJUNCTS — OPA · NPA · Two-Person BMV (SEAL)

Simple manoeuvres FIRST: Head tilt–chin lift (jaw thrust if trauma). Suction MUST be ready before any adjunct.

Contraindications: OPA in conscious patient (gag intact) = instant fail · NPA in basal skull fracture (raccoon eyes, Battle's sign, CSF leak) = absolute contraindication

Adjunct	Indication + Sizing	Key Script
OPA	GCS ≤8, unconscious, NO gag reflex. Size: corner of mouth to angle of mandible.	"Unconscious, GCS ≤8, no gag. Sizing OPA. Following natural curvature. Suction ready."
NPA	Semi-conscious, intact gag. Size: little finger width at nostril. NO skull fracture.	"No skull fracture signs. Sizing NPA — little finger. Lubricating. Bevel to nasal septum."

Two-Person BMV — SEAL:

S=Seal (C-E grip) · E=Elevate jaw into mask · A=Assist (colleague squeezes 10–12/min over 1 sec) · L=Look for chest rise

"C-E grip maintained. Colleague delivers slow breaths — watching visible chest rise. If BMV fails ×2 attempts → call senior."

Suction on withdrawal: Apply suction ONLY on withdrawal, NOT insertion. <10 seconds per pass. Hyperoxygenate before and after.

OXYGEN THERAPY — O_2 SAFE · Device Selection

Targets: 94–98% most acutely ill · 88–92% stable COPD/at risk of hypercapnia (pending ABG)
Always: Prescribe on drug chart with TARGET SATURATION RANGE documented

Device	When to Use	Key Safety
Nasal cannulae 1–4 L/min	Mild hypoxia, stable	Low-flow only · allows eating/talking
Simple face mask 5–10 L/min	Moderate hypoxia	Must be ≥5 L/min to prevent CO_2 rebreathing
Venturi mask	STABLE COPD — colour-coded jet sets FiO_2	Read jet colour carefully · target 88–92%
Non-rebreathe mask 15 L/min	Severe hypoxia	Fill reservoir bag BEFORE application · target 94–98%

O_2 SAFE: O=Target (94-98%/88-92%) · 2=Device (Venturi for COPD) · S=Flow appropriate · A=Assess response (SpO_2+ABG) · F=Follow-up/escalate · E=Evaluate for NIV (COPD acidotic+conscious)
COPD script: "Controlled O_2, Venturi mask. If peri-arrest or critically hypoxic → high-flow initially, then titrate once ABG available."

CHEST DRAINS — LAT · WISE · SWAB · SUCTION

LAT — Triangle of Safety: Lateral border of pectoralis major · Anterior border of latissimus dorsi · 5th ICS mid-axillary line
Safety Rules: System BELOW chest ALWAYS · NEVER clamp without senior instruction · NEVER milk or strip
Dislodged drain: Occlusive dressing + call senior immediately. DO NOT reinsert.

WISE — Primary Drain Monitoring:
W=Water seal (fluid level correct) · I=Intercostal site (erythema, emphysema) · S=Swinging (with respiration = patent) · E=Effective drainage (intermittent bubbling = normal)
Script: "Water seal correct, site clean, swinging with respiration — drain patent, effective drainage."

SWAB — Daily Check:
S=Suction (on/off level?) · W=Water level (correct?) · A=Air leak (continuous bubbles = system leak — check connections) · B=Bubbling (intermittent with cough only = normal)

Finding	Meaning	Action
Swinging with respiration	Drain patent — lung moving	Normal — document

Finding	Meaning	Action
Swinging stops	Blockage/kink OR full expansion	Check clinically + senior review
Continuous bubbling	System leak / ongoing air leak	Check ALL connections immediately
Bubbling stops (pneumothorax drain)	Pneumothorax resolved	Consider removal criteria
No swinging + respiratory distress	Blocked/tension	Senior review · prepare decompression

SUCTION — Removal Criteria:
Swinging stopped · Unremarkable breath sounds · CXR confirms full re-expansion · Time (output <100mL/24h) · Inspiration hold/Valsalva · Occlusive dressing immediately · New CXR post-removal

Escalate Immediately If:

Persistent hypoxia despite O_2 · COPD patient drowsy (CO_2 retention) · GCS dropping · Tension pneumothorax suspected · Drain dislodged · Massive air leak · >2 failed attempts
"This patient is deteriorating. Calling for senior help immediately and staying until they arrive."
Tension pneumothorax: "O_2 must NOT delay immediate needle decompression. Call senior. 2nd ICS MCL or 4th/5th ICS anterior axillary line."

Examiner Checklist

Airway + Oxygen ✓	Chest Drain ✓
✓ ABCDE approach used	✓ LAT triangle of safety confirmed
✓ Suction ready before any adjunct	✓ System below chest level
✓ Simple manoeuvres first	✓ WISE monitoring completed
✓ OPA: GCS ≤8 + no gag confirmed	✓ SWAB daily check done
✓ NPA: skull fracture excluded	✓ No clamping without senior instruction
✓ Two-person BMV with SEAL	✓ Continuous bubbling: checked connections
✓ Correct O_2 device for context	✓ SUCTION removal criteria reviewed
✓ Venturi for stable COPD	✓ Dislodgement: occlusive dressing + senior
✓ Target SpO_2 on drug chart	✓ Escalated if deteriorating
✓ SpO_2 reassessed after oxygen	✓ Patient advised + documented

Final Exam Mantra

AIRWAY: ABCDE → look/listen/feel → suction ready → OPA (GCS≤8, no gag) · NPA (semi-conscious, no skull Fx) · 2-person BMV (SEAL)

OXYGEN = DRUG: prescribe on chart with TARGET · Venturi COPD 88–92% · NRM severe hypoxia (fill bag first) · reassess within minutes

DRAIN: WISE + SWAB + LAT · below chest ALWAYS · NEVER clamp without senior · SUCTION removal criteria

Escalate: COPD drowsy · GCS dropping · tension pneumothorax · drain dislodged · >2 failed attempts

Gold Closing:
"ABCDE used. OPA [sized/inserted] / NPA [sized/inserted] / BMV [SEAL, 2-person, chest rise]. O_2 device: [appropriate]. Prescribed on chart with target [94-98%/88-92%]. Drain: WISE check normal, SWAB: no continuous leak, system below chest. Never clamped. Escalated if deteriorating."

COPD = Venturi 88-92% pending ABG	OPA GCS ≤8 unconscious + no gag	NPA no skull Fx semi-conscious only	2-person BMV SEAL mnemonic always	Suction ready before any adjunct
Fill NRM bag first before application	Drain below chest always non-negotiable	Never clamp without senior instruction	Continuous bubbling check connections now	O2 = drug prescribe with target on chart

TOP 5 EXAMINER Q&A · AIRWAY ADJUNCTS, OXYGEN & CHEST DRAINS	
Q1. Sizing an oropharyngeal airway?	Incisors to angle of the jaw; insert inverted and rotate (adult): if the gag reflex is present, it does not stay.
Q2. When is an NPA contraindicated?	Suspected base-of-skull fracture: choose an OPA or escalate to advanced airway support.
Q3. Bag-valve-mask failing to ventilate?	Optimise: two-person technique, airway manoeuvres, adjunct in place, check the seal: then call for airway expertise.
Q4. Oxygen prescription essentials?	Device, flow rate, and a documented target saturation range: 94–98% standard, 88–92% in CO2-retention risk.
Q5. Chest drain safe zone?	The triangle of safety: anterior to mid-axillary line, above the 5th intercostal space, going above the rib below.
CURVEBALL	The drain is swinging but suddenly stops after movement. Check the tubing for kinks and the drain position before assuming resolution: a blocked drain on a tension chest kills.

CHAPTER 67 · THE PRESCRIBING CONSULTATION & CORE CALCULATIONS

SAFE PRESCRIBE · ORIP · IOAPM · 5 Rs · Calculations · CD Rules · Oxygen · Stewardship

CORE · CAUTION — INSTANT FAIL RISK · DRUG CHART · CALCULATIONS · PATIENT SAFETY

Abbreviations used in this chapter: **BNF** British National Formulary · **COPD** Chronic Obstructive Pulmonary Disease · **HF** Heart Failure · **NBM** Nil By Mouth · **NKDA** No Known Drug Allergies · **NSAID** Non-Steroidal Anti-Inflammatory Drug

DISTINCTION — Golden Triad of Prescribing Fail — INSTANT FAIL, No Exceptions: 1. Don't ask about/document allergies · 2. Decimal error (.5 mg instead of 0.5 mg) · 3. Controlled drug in figures only

INSTANT FAILS: No allergy · Decimal error · PRN without interval · CD figures only · Wrong chart section · No signature · No renal check · No indication (antibiotics) · Ignore drug interaction

SAY — Golden Rule: "Allergy first, BNF always, show your working, sign and date. If you would not give it to your own family member — stop and check."

SAFE PRESCRIBE — Master Framework

S	Status	Check obs, NEWS, recent labs: eGFR, U&Es
A	Allergy ← FIRST	"Any drug allergies?" → document NKDA or specific allergy
F	Function (renal/hepatic)	eGFR check · dose adjustment · drug interactions
E	Existing meds	"What medications do you take? When was last dose?"
P	Precise drug (generic)	Paracetamol NOT Panadol — NHS standard
R	Route	PO / IV / IM / SC / PR / inhaler / NG
E	Exact dose (BNF)	BNF-checked · calculation shown · decimal-safe
S	Schedule	Frequency · PRN interval · maximum dose
C	Clear documentation	Correct section (ORIP) · legible · no unsafe abbreviations
R	Review plan	Review U&Es/fluids in 24h · stop date
I	Indication	Document reason — mandatory for antibiotics
B	BNF check	Dose · contraindications · interactions · renal adjustment
E	End with signature	Sign · print name · date · GMC/bleep

Safety Rules — Decimal · Abbreviations · ORIP · PRN

Decimal Safety: ✗ .5 mg ✓ 0.5 mg · ✗ 5.0 mg ✓ 5 mg — Leading zero, no trailing zeros. ".5 can be misread as 5 mg = 10× overdose"

Unsafe Abbreviations: ✗ U (misread as 0) → write "units" · ✗ IU (misread as IV) → write "international units" · ✗ µg (misread as mg) → write "mcg"

ORIP Section	Use	Example
Once Only (O)	Single/STAT dose	Co-amoxiclav IV STAT pre-op
Regular (R)	Daily scheduled meds	Amlodipine 5mg OD
IV Fluids (I)	Fluids with rate	NaCl 0.9% 1L over 8 hours = 125 mL/hr
PRN (P)	As required + RIM	Morphine SC PRN 4–6 hourly · max dose stated

PRN — RIM Framework: R=Reason ("for pain") · I=Interval (minimum time: "4–6 hourly") · M=Maximum ("max 4g/24h")

Core Calculations — Always Show Working Aloud

Type	Formula	Example
Weight-based	Dose = weight (kg) × mg/kg	"70 kg × dose/kg from BNF = [X] mg"
Infusion rate	mL/hr = volume (mL) ÷ time (hours)	"1000 mL ÷ 8 hours = 125 mL/hr"
Oral liquid	Volume = (required ÷ stock strength) × volume	"300 mg needed, stock 250mg/5mL = 6 mL"

High-Risk Drugs — IOAPM:
I=Insulin (never "U") · O=Opioids (monitor RR) · A=Anticoagulants (check platelets/eGFR) · P=Potassium IV (NEVER bolus) · M=Methotrexate (ONCE WEEKLY not daily)

Controlled Drugs — SAFE:
S=Signature (own handwriting) · A=All details (dose in WORDS + FIGURES: "Ten (10) mg") · F=Formulation specific · E=Endorse quantity (discharge only)

5 Rs — Final Check Before Handing Over: Right patient · Right drug · Right dose · Right route · Right time

IV Fluids · Oxygen · Antibiotic Stewardship

IV Fluids — Always State: Why (maintenance/replacement/resuscitation) · What · How much · How fast · When review

Script: "1L of 0.18% NaCl / 4% glucose with 40 mmol KCl over 12h (~85 mL/hr) — for maintenance (NBM), per NICE NG29 (≈25–30 mL/kg/day). Review U&Es + fluid balance in 24h."

Caution: Heart failure · renal impairment · elderly · pulmonary oedema risk

Oxygen — It Is a Drug:
Most patients: target SpO_2 94–98% · COPD/at-risk: 88–92% (prevents CO_2 retention)
"Oxygen via nasal cannulae — target SpO_2 94–98%. Review sats + ABG in 1 hour."

Antibiotic Stewardship: Document indication · Review/stop date · Avoid viral illness · Check penicillin allergy · "This is viral — antibiotics not indicated."

THINK — Special Populations · Analgesia Ladder

Group	Must Check + Script
Elderly / frail	"Start low, go slow — elderly: lower dose, monitor carefully."
Renal (eGFR <30)	"eGFR [X] — BNF dose adjustment. Avoiding NSAIDs, metformin, nitrofurantoin."
Hepatic impairment	"Avoiding paracetamol in severe hepatic disease. Checking hepatotoxic drugs."
Pregnancy	"Pregnant — checking BNF pregnancy section. Avoiding ACE inhibitors, tetracyclines, NSAIDs (3rd trimester)."
Polypharmacy	"Multiple meds — checking warfarin/DOACs/lithium interactions."

WHO Analgesia Ladder:
Step 1: Paracetamol (max 4g/24h) · Step 2: NSAID (avoid eGFR <30, GI bleed, HF) · Step 3: Weak opioid (codeine) · Step 4: Strong opioid (morphine — monitor RR, avoid renal failure)

SAY — Patient Explanation Scripts

Antibiotics: "For your infection. Take the full course. Side effects: diarrhoea, rash. Seek help if breathing difficulty or facial swelling."

Opioids: "Strong painkiller. May cause drowsiness, constipation. Don't drive. Seek help if unusually sleepy or difficulty breathing."

NSAIDs: "For pain and inflammation. Take with food. Seek help if black stools or severe stomach pain. Kidneys checked."

Methotrexate: "ONCE WEEKLY — not daily. I'll repeat: ONCE A WEEK. Bloods monitored regularly."

Anticoagulants: "Thins blood to prevent clots. Easy bruising. Seek help immediately if unusual bleeding, black stools, or fall."

Examiner Checklist

Prescribing ✓	Safety + Communication ✓
✓ Allergy asked + documented first	✓ Indication documented (antibiotics)
✓ eGFR/renal function checked	✓ Review plan + stop date stated
✓ Drug interactions checked	✓ 5 Rs completed before handover
✓ Generic name used	✓ CD: words + figures + own signature
✓ BNF dose confirmed	✓ PRN: reason + interval + max dose (RIM)
✓ Calculation shown aloud	✓ ORIP: correct section chosen
✓ Decimal-safe (0.5 not .5)	✓ Patient: indication + SE + red flags
✓ No unsafe abbreviations	✓ Escalation plan if deterioration

Final Exam Mantra

SAFE PRESCRIBE: Status · Allergy(FIRST) · Function · Existing → Precise · Route · Exact · Schedule · Clear · Review · Indication · BNF · End/sign

ORIP: Once · Regular · IV · PRN · PRN-RIM: Reason · Interval · Maximum

IOAPM high-risk: Insulin · Opioids · Anticoagulants · Potassium IV · Methotrexate (once weekly)

CD SAFE: Signature · All details (words+figures) · Formulation · Endorse

5 Rs: Right patient · drug · dose · route · time · Oxygen: 94–98% (88–92% COPD)

Gold Closing:

"Allergy confirmed (NKDA). eGFR checked. BNF dose confirmed. Calculation: [X]. Decimal-safe: [0.5 not .5]. ORIP section: [correct]. Generic name. Indication documented. PRN: reason, interval, max. CD: words + figures + signed. 5 Rs complete. Review in 24h. Explained to patient: indication, side effects, red flags."

Allergy first every station always	0.5 not .5 leading zero rule	CD words + figures "Ten (10) mg"	ORIP sections right section = valid	PRN = RIM reason interval max
5 Rs final check before handover	IOAPM caution insulin to methotrexate	BNF always never memorise doses	Indication documented antibiotics mandatory	eGFR before prescribing renal dose adjust

TOP 5 EXAMINER Q&A · PRESCRIBING CONSULTATION & CALCULATIONS

Q1. The non-negotiables before any prescription?	Allergies asked and documented, identity, weight where relevant, renal/hepatic function, interactions, and pregnancy status.

TOP 5 EXAMINER Q&A · PRESCRIBING CONSULTATION & CALCULATIONS	
Q2. How do you verbalise a dose calculation?	State the formula, the numbers, and the units at each step: then sanity-check the answer aloud against a sensible range.
Q3. Where do you put the decimal point rules?	Never a trailing zero (5 mg, not 5.0 mg): always a leading zero (0.5 mg, not .5 mg): micrograms written in full.
Q4. The patient asks "is this safe?"	Answer honestly: main benefits, common and serious side effects, what to do if they occur: then check understanding.
Q5. What closes a prescribing station?	Signature-level details: drug, dose, route, frequency, duration, indication documented: plus monitoring and review plan.
CURVEBALL	Your calculated dose feels too large. Trust the discomfort: recheck units and weight, state you would confirm against the BNF and with a colleague: the pause is the pass.

CHAPTER 68 · PRESCRIBING SAFETY: HIGH-RISK DRUGS & COMMON ERRORS

WILM NOSABDG · PINK · FAB · TAC · CANS · STOP · CARE · ACE-RISK · TEACH-BACK

CORE · HIGH YIELD · CAUTION — INSTANT FAIL RISK · Every Prescribing Station

Abbreviations used in this chapter: **CKD** Chronic Kidney Disease · **HF** Heart Failure · **ICH** Intracranial Haemorrhage · **MTX** Methotrexate · **NKDA** No Known Drug Allergies · **NSAID** Non-Steroidal Anti-Inflammatory Drug · **PCC** Prothrombin Complex Concentrate · **PPI** Proton Pump Inhibitor

DISTINCTION — Golden Triad of Fail:

1. MTX prescribed DAILY (must be ONCE WEEKLY — daily can be fatal)
2. Insulin written as "u" (must be "units" in full)
3. Warfarin major bleed reversed with Vitamin K alone (need PCC + Vitamin K)

INSTANT FAILS: No allergy check · No monitoring arranged · No counselling/teach-back · Missing renal impairment · Ignoring drug interactions

SAY — First Question: "Is this patient stable? Any allergies?" — Safety first before prescribing anything.

WILM NOSABDG: W=Warfarin · I=Insulin · L=Lithium · M=Methotrexate · N=NSAIDs · O=Opioids · S=Steroids · A=ACE inhibitors · B=Beta-blockers · D=Digoxin · G=Gentamicin

1. Anticoagulants · MTX · Lithium

Warfarin — PINK Reversal:

P=Pressing emergency (major bleed/ICH) → PCC + IV Vitamin K · I=Intermediate → assess severity · N=No rush (high INR, no bleeding) → oral Vitamin K · K=Keep in mind: PCC works immediately

Key interactions: Antibiotics ↑INR · Amiodarone ↑INR · Cranberry ↑INR · NSAIDs ↑bleed risk · Rifampicin/Carbamazepine ↓INR

Methotrexate — ONCE WEEKLY (NEVER DAILY — FATAL):

"The most important thing: take this ONCE A WEEK on the same day. Taking it DAILY can be fatal."

FAB Monitoring: F=Folic acid (different day) · A=Avoid trimethoprim · B=Bloods (FBC, LFTs, U&Es)

STOP MTX if: Mouth ulcers · sore throat · fever · bruising · breathlessness · rash → seek urgent help

Lithium — TAC Toxicity:

T=Tremor (coarse) · A=Ataxia (slurred speech) · C=Confusion/drowsiness

Monitoring: After dose change → level at 1 week then weekly until stable. Stable patient → every 3 months. Renal + thyroid every 6–12 months.

Red flags → check levels urgently: New diarrhoea/vomiting · polyuria · slurred speech · worsening tremor · confusion

2. Insulin · Steroids · NSAIDs · Opioids

Insulin: NEVER write "u" or "U" — always write "units" in full (prevents 10× dosing error)
Basal: Glargine/Detemir — once/twice daily, fixed time. Bolus: Novorapid/Actrapid — with meals
Hypo: Fast-acting sugar → recheck glucose after 15 min. Signs: sweating, shaking, hunger, confusion, palpitations

Drug	Mnemonic + Key Points	Must Say
Steroids	CARE: Cover PPI · Adrenal suppression (never stop abruptly) · Raised glucose · Exacerbates infection. Long-term >3m: bisphosphonates.	"Taper slowly. Sick-day rules. Monitor glucose."
NSAIDs	CANS: CKD · Asthma (aspirin-sensitive) · No if dehydrated · Stomach ulcer/history. Avoid 3rd trimester.	"Contraindicated if CKD/asthma/3rd trimester."
Opioids	STOP: Sedation (monitor RR) · Titrate (start low) · Opioid naive (reduce) · Prescribe laxatives ALWAYS	"Laxatives always. Seek help: RR <8, pinpoint pupils, drowsy."

3. Cardiovascular · Psychotropics

Drug	Key Points
ACE inhibitors	ACE-RISK: Avoid pregnancy · Check creatinine · Electrolytes (K+) · Renal artery stenosis contraindicated · Initial hypotension (bedtime) · Stop angioedema · K+ rises. Sick-day rules: stop if vomiting/diarrhoea/dehydrated.
Beta-blockers	BBLOCK: Bradycardia (avoid HR <50) · Bronchospasm (avoid asthma) · Low BP · Observe fatigue · Contraindicated acute HF · Keep from hypo-unawareness
Digoxin	DIG: Dose reduce in renal impairment · Interactions (amiodarone, verapamil ↑levels) · Gum toxicity (nausea, yellow vision, arrhythmias) → check levels
Gentamicin	ONCE: Once daily · Need levels (pre + post dose) · Creatinine check · Eight mg/kg weight-based. Toxicity: nephrotoxicity + ototoxicity
SSRIs	SEROTONIN: Early activation (monitor suicide risk first 2 weeks in young) · No abrupt stop (taper slowly) · Sexual side effects · Nausea (take with food) · Serotonin syndrome risk
Antipsychotics	NMS-QT-MET: Neuroleptic Malignant Syndrome · QT prolongation (ECG if risk) · Metabolic syndrome (weight, glucose, lipids)

Sick-Day Rules · Pregnancy · Stewardship · Deprescribing

Sick-Day Rules (if vomiting/diarrhoea/dehydrated):
STOP: ACE inhibitors · ARBs · NSAIDs · diuretics · metformin · Restart when eating and drinking normally

Avoid in Pregnancy	Status
Warfarin	AVOID — teratogenic
ACE inhibitors	AVOID — renal agenesis
Methotrexate	AVOID — teratogenic
NSAIDs (3rd trimester)	AVOID — premature ductus closure
Statins	AVOID
Lithium	CAUTION — Ebstein anomaly
Beta-blockers	Labetalol OK — monitor growth

Antibiotic Stewardship — STEWARD: Spectrum (narrowest) · Time (shortest) · Evidence (confirm infection) · Watch (review 48h) · Allergy (clarify reaction) · Renal (dose adjust) · Document
Allergy clarification: "Was it a rash, swelling, or difficulty breathing?" (rash ≠ anaphylaxis)

Deprescribing — STOP & THINK: Still indicated? · Time-limited? · Overlapping drugs? · Patient preference? · Harm vs benefit?
Elderly caution: Start low, go slow · Avoid sedatives + anticholinergics · Review benzodiazepines, PPIs, opioids, anticholinergics

SAY — TEACH-BACK · Examiner Trap Recognition

TEACH-BACK — Use After Every Counselling:
Tell (how to take) · Explain (indication) · Ask ("Tell me how you'll take this") · Check understanding · Highlight red flags · Back (written info) · Arrange monitoring
"Tell me how you'll take your methotrexate." · "What will you do if you notice bleeding?" (warfarin) · "What signs make you seek urgent help?" (opioids)

Examiner Trap	Say This
Daily MTX on chart	"Must be ONCE WEEKLY — daily can be fatal."
Insulin "u"	"Writing 'units' in full — prevents 10× dosing error."
Warfarin + antibiotics	"Check INR in 2–3 days — antibiotics increase warfarin effect."
NSAID + asthma	"Contraindicated — aspirin-sensitive asthma — using alternative."
Warfarin major bleed	"PCC immediately PLUS Vitamin K — not Vitamin K alone."
Lithium without monitoring	"Lithium requires regular level monitoring — arranging this."
Digoxin + renal impairment	"Dose adjust — checking eGFR first."

Examiner Checklist

Drug Safety ✓	Counselling + Documentation ✓
✓ Allergy asked + documented first	✓ TEACH-BACK used
✓ Renal function checked	✓ Indication documented
✓ Drug interactions checked	✓ Monitoring arranged
✓ MTX: once weekly confirmed	✓ Sick-day rules given if appropriate
✓ Insulin: "units" in full	✓ Pregnancy safety checked
✓ Warfarin: PINK reversal known	✓ Written information offered
✓ Lithium: TAC toxicity + levels	✓ Safety-net: when to seek help
✓ Opioids: laxatives prescribed	✓ Review date documented
✓ QT drugs: ECG if risk	✓ Escalation if emergency

Final Exam Mantra

WILM NOSABDG: W=Warfarin(PINK) · I=Insulin(never u) · L=Lithium(TAC) · M=MTX(ONCE WEEKLY)

N=NSAIDs(CANS) · O=Opioids(STOP+laxatives) · S=Steroids(CARE+taper) · A=ACE-i(ACE-RISK)

B=Beta-blockers(BBLOCK) · D=Digoxin(DIG) · G=Gentamicin(ONCE levels renal)

Sick-day: stop ACEi/ARBs/NSAIDs/diuretics/metformin if vomiting · Pregnancy: avoid warfarin/ACEi/MTX/NSAIDs/statins

TEACH-BACK always · STEWARD antibiotics · STOP & THINK deprescribing

Gold Closing:

"Prescribed [drug] at [dose] [frequency]. Allergies checked (NKDA). Contraindications: renal, pregnancy, interactions — all clear. Monitoring arranged: [bloods/levels/follow-up]. Counselled with teach-back — patient confirms understanding. Written instructions given. Safety-net: seek urgent help if [specific signs]. Documented clearly."

MTX once weekly never daily = fatal	Insulin = "units" never "u" ever	Warfarin bleed PCC + Vitamin K	Lithium TAC tremor ataxia confusion	NSAIDs = CANS CKD asthma 3rd trim
Opioids = laxatives always co-prescribe	Steroids = taper never stop abruptly	ACE sick-day stop if vomiting/diarrhoea	TEACH-BACK check understanding	QT drugs ECG if risk factors

TOP 5 EXAMINER Q&A · PRESCRIBING SAFETY: HIGH-RISK DRUGS	
Q1. The classic high-risk drug groups?	Anticoagulants, insulin, opioids, methotrexate, gentamicin/vancomycin, potassium, chemotherapy: each needs specific checks.
Q2. Methotrexate's fatal error?	Daily instead of weekly dosing: always state the weekly day and co-prescribed folic acid: never co-prescribe trimethoprim.
Q3. Insulin's writing rule?	The word "units" in full, never "U": and never abbreviate insulin names.
Q4. Gentamicin essentials?	Dose by weight and renal function, levels per protocol, and stop/adjust based on them: nephro- and ototoxicity stated.
Q5. Warfarin interactions you must volunteer?	Antibiotics (especially macrolides), NSAIDs, amiodarone, alcohol: check INR more often around any change.
CURVEBALL	A senior's verbal order sounds wrong. Politely verify before giving: read back the drug, dose and route, and check the BNF together: hierarchy never overrides safety.

CHAPTER 69 · THINKING ALOUD: THE CLINICAL REASONING TECHNIQUE EXAMINERS SCORE

Explicit Reasoning · Structured Differentials · Visible Thinking · Markable Steps

CORE · HIGH YIELD · Every Station

Abbreviations used in this chapter: **PE** Pulmonary Embolism

DISTINCTION — Golden Rule: "If it's in your head, say it out loud."
Examiners score your REASONING, not just your answer. Silent thinking = invisible reasoning = no marks.
High-Risk Behaviours: Unsignposted silence >10 seconds · Diagnoses without justification · Tests without "because" · Data dump (no synthesis) · No safety net · Missing life-threatening differential

SAY — Blueprint: GATHER → ORGANISE → PRIORITISE → JUSTIFY → SYNTHESISE → PLAN → SAFETY NET
"Say what you think → Say why → Say what next. The examiner's silent question: Would I trust this candidate alone?"

THINK — Five Core Steps — What Examiners Want to Hear

Step 1: Most Likely	"The most likely diagnosis is [X] because [Y]." — Always lead with common things.
Step 2: Life-Threatening	"I must not miss [red flag condition] because [risk]." — State this regardless of age or context.
Step 3: Justify Tests	"I would request [test] because I'm looking for [finding], which would confirm/exclude [diagnosis] and change management."
Step 4: Synthesise (SIPS)	S=Synthesise the finding · I=Interpret · P=Prioritise in context · S=Signpost next step. "Putting this together, the pattern fits [X]."
Step 5: Escalate + Safety Net	"If they deteriorate, I will escalate to senior." — "I'll advise them to return if [criteria]."

Golden 30 Seconds · 3-Tier Differential · BECAUSE Rule

Golden 30 Seconds — After History (aim by minute 3–4):
1. "Let me organise my thoughts…" (signpost the pause)
2. "The most likely diagnosis is [X] because [Y]."
3. "I must not miss [life-threatening differential]."
4. "The safest next step is [action] because [reason]."

Tier	Focus	Example
1. Most Likely	Common things first	"Given fever and cough, pneumonia is most likely."
2. Life-Threatening	Red flags, dangerous mimics	"I must not miss PE due to pleuritic pain."
3. Other Possibilities	Keep in mind	"I should also consider malignancy in smokers."

BECAUSE Rule: Never order a test without saying why.
"I would request [test] because I'm looking for [finding], which would confirm or exclude [diagnosis] and change management."
Time-critical: "This needs urgent investigation because delay increases risk of [complication]."

THINK — Cognitive Bias Traps · Updating Reasoning

Bias	OSCE Example	How to Avoid
Anchoring	"Young patient can't have MI"	Always state must-not-miss regardless of age
Premature closure	Stop thinking after first fit diagnosis	State alternatives after leading diagnosis
Confirmation bias	Only ask questions supporting your hunch	"What makes this NOT pneumonia?" — disconfirming questions
Availability bias	Availability bias: last memorable case biases current diagnosis — "I just saw a PE so everything is a PE". Reset: "What is most likely for THIS patient, not what I saw most recently?"	Use a hierarchical differential anchored to this patient's findings, not your most recent memorable case. Actively ask: "If I had NOT just seen that PE, what would my differential be?"

Updating your differential aloud scores highly:
"Initially I thought pneumonia. However, normal chest examination makes PE more likely now."
"This result changes my thinking. Pneumonia is now less likely; I'm concerned about PE."
To avoid anchoring: "I want to avoid anchoring — although pneumonia is most likely, I'm keeping PE in mind."

Handling Uncertainty · OSCE Traps · When Stuck

Situation	Script
Need to pause	"Let me organise my thoughts…"

Situation	Script
Unsure of diagnosis	"I'm not 100% sure. Pattern fits [X] best, but I must rule out [Y]. Next step is [test] because…"
Patient asks your opinion	"At this stage, most likely is [X]. However, I must rule out [Y]."
Examiner challenges you	"That's a good point — let me explain how I'm thinking about it."
You realise you missed something	"Let me correct that — actually, the most likely is…"
Time pressure	"I'll summarise my key findings and outline my plan."
Stuck completely	Signpost → state most likely → state life-threat → pick safest next step + justify it

Special Station Scripts:
Emergency: "Airway patent, breathing compromised — oxygen before diagnostics."
Paediatrics: "Must consider safeguarding given the presentation."
Psychiatry: "Assessing risk to self, others, and vulnerability."
Conflicting info: "When symptoms conflict, I prioritise red flags over typical features."

Weak vs Strong Answer — Worked Example

✗ **Weak:** "It's pneumonia. I'll do CXR." — No reasoning. No differential. No justification. No safety net.

✓ **Strong:**
"Let me organise my thoughts. Most likely is pneumonia because of fever, cough, and focal chest signs. I must not miss PE given the pleuritic pain."
"I would request CXR because I'm looking for consolidation, which would confirm pneumonia and guide antibiotic therapy."
"Putting this together, the pattern fits pneumonia. My plan: start antibiotics and monitor. If they deteriorate, I'll escalate. Advise return if symptoms worsen."
Why it passes: Clear structure · Visible reasoning · Justification · Synthesis · Safety net

Examiner Checklist — Every Station

Reasoning ✓	Safety + Communication ✓
✓ No unsignposted silence >10 seconds	✓ Life-threatening differential named
✓ Golden 30 seconds delivered	✓ Safety net verbalised
✓ Most likely + "because"	✓ Escalation plan stated
✓ BECAUSE rule for every test	✓ Differential updated after new findings
✓ SIPS synthesis used	✓ Cognitive bias avoided (anchoring stated)

Reasoning ✓	Safety + Communication ✓
✓ 3-tier differential given	✓ Recovery phrase used if stuck
✓ Tone conversational (not scripted)	✓ Correction made openly if needed

Final Exam Mantra

Five Core Steps: Most likely (because) · Must-not-miss · Justify tests (because) · SIPS synthesis · Escalate + safety net

Golden 30 Seconds: "Let me organise my thoughts… Most likely is [X] because… I must not miss… Safest next step…"

3-Tier Differential: Most likely → Life-threatening → Other possibilities

SIPS: Synthesise · Interpret · Prioritise · Signpost — never data dump

Update reasoning aloud · State biases · Correct openly · Safety net always

Gold Closing:

"Most likely is [X] because [Y]. I must not miss [life-threat]. I would request [test] because it would change management. Putting this together, the pattern fits [X]. My plan: [management]. If they deteriorate, I'll escalate. Return if [safety net criteria]."

"If in head say it" golden rule always	Signpost pauses not silence = marks	Most likely + because every time	Must not miss life-threat always	BECAUSE for tests what AND why
SIPS synthesis not data dump	3-tier differential structured not random	Update aloud dynamic reasoning	State biases anchoring avoided	Safety net always never just discharge

TOP 5 EXAMINER Q&A · THINKING ALOUD: CLINICAL REASONING	
Q1. Why does thinking aloud score?	Examiners mark visible reasoning: silent excellence reads as absence: name what you see, what it means, what you will do.
Q2. The structure of a spoken differential?	Most likely, most dangerous, and the discriminating features you will use: in that order, out loud.
Q3. How do you voice uncertainty safely?	"The picture is not yet clear: the possibilities are X and Y: the safest path while we clarify is Z".
Q4. Anchoring: how do you show you avoid it?	Verbally revisit: "the new finding does not fit my working diagnosis: I am broadening the differential".
Q5. Closing the loop aloud?	After every action: state the expected response, the reassessment, and the trigger for escalation.
CURVEBALL	You realise mid-station your initial diagnosis was wrong. Say so: "I am revising my impression because of X": examiners reward the correction more than the original error costs.

CHAPTER 70 · ECG & ABG INTERPRETATION

KILL · RRAIS · AIL · BAD · ROME · WINTER · WIDE

CORE · CAUTION — INSTANT FAIL RISK · A&E · AMU · Cardiology · Resp · ICU

Abbreviations used in this chapter: **CHB** Complete Heart Block · **COPD** Chronic Obstructive Pulmonary Disease · **DKA** Diabetic Ketoacidosis · **GTN** Glyceryl Trinitrate · **LBBB** Left Bundle Branch Block · **NIV** Non-Invasive Ventilation · **NSTEMI** Non-ST-Elevation Myocardial Infarction · **PCI** Percutaneous Coronary Intervention · **PE** Pulmonary Embolism · **STEMI** ST-Elevation Myocardial Infarction · **SVT** Supraventricular Tachycardia · **VF** Ventricular Fibrillation · **VT** Ventricular Tachycardia

DISTINCTION — ECG — 4 INSTANT FAILS:
STEMI (immediate reperfusion) · VT unstable (shock) / stable (amiodarone) · Complete heart block (pacing) · Hyperkalaemia (peaked T → wide QRS → sine wave → IV calcium)
DISTINCTION — ABG — 4 INSTANT FAILS:
pH <7.2 or >7.6 (ICU review) · PaO_2 <8 kPa (oxygen) · $PaCO_2$ >6.5 + acidosis (NIV/ventilation) · K+ <2.5 or >6.5 (urgent correction)
STOP and ACT. Do not continue systematic interpretation without flagging the emergency.

SAY — Meta-Framework: SCAN → SYSTEMATIC → CORRELATE → ACT → ESCALATE
Danger First · KILL/BAD scan · RRAIS/5-Step · Link to scenario · Treat · Senior/ICU

ECG — KILL First-Look · RRAIS Systematic

KILL — 5-Second Scan (do FIRST):
K=K^+ changes (peaked T, wide QRS, sine wave) · I=Ischaemia (ST elevation/depression) · L=Lethal rhythms (VT/VF/Torsades — polymorphic VT with prolonged QTc) · L=Low rate (complete heart block) CAUTION — Calcium distinction: gluconate 10% (hyperkalaemia — give IV) ≠ chloride 10% (cardiac arrest only — 3× elemental Ca). Do NOT substitute.
"First, I'll scan for life-threatening findings using KILL — no K^+ changes, no ischaemia, no lethal rhythms, no low rate."

	Step	Normal	Abnormal / Verbalisation
R	Rate	60–100 bpm	Tachy >100 (300÷large squares, regular) · Brady <60 (6-sec×10, irregular)
R	Rhythm	Regular	AF = irregularly irregular · Flutter = regular sawtooth · Regularly irregular = 2nd degree HB
A	Axis	I↑ aVF↑ = normal	I↑ aVF↓ = LAD (LVH/LBBB/inf MI) · I↓ aVF↑ = RAD (RVH/PE/COPD)
I	Intervals	PR 0.12–0.20s, QRS <0.12s, QTc <0.45s	PR >0.20 = 1° HB · CHB = no P-QRS relation · Wide QRS = BBB/VT · QTc >0.45 = torsades risk
S	ST changes	Isoelectric	Elevation = STEMI/pericarditis · Depression = ischaemia/NSTEMI

PR Interval: Progressively lengthening + dropped = Mobitz I · Constant PR + intermittent dropped = Mobitz II (risk of CHB) · No P-QRS relation = Complete Heart Block → PACING

LBBB + chest pain = STEMI equivalent until proven otherwise. Broad complex tachycardia = VT until proven otherwise.

STEMI Locations (AIL) · Special Patterns · ST Elevation Traps

Location	Leads	Verbalisation
Anterior	V1–V4	"ST elevation V1–V4 — anterior STEMI — immediate reperfusion."
Inferior	II, III, aVF	"ST elevation II, III, aVF — inferior STEMI."
Lateral	I, aVL, V5–V6	"ST elevation I, aVL, V5–V6 — lateral STEMI."

Special Patterns — Don't Miss:

Pericarditis: Diffuse saddle-shaped ST elevation + PR depression (no reciprocal changes)

Wellens syndrome: Biphasic/inverted T waves V2–V3 → critical LAD stenosis → URGENT angiogram

De Winter T waves: Upsloping ST depression + peaked T V2–V4 → proximal LAD occlusion → treat as STEMI

Posterior MI: ST depression V1–V3 + tall R waves → treat as STEMI

ECG Emergencies — Act Immediately

Emergency Finding	Immediate Action
STEMI	Aspirin · O_2 if SpO_2 <94% · morphine · GTN · immediate reperfusion (PCI or thrombolysis)
VT (unstable)	DC cardioversion immediately
VT (stable)	IV amiodarone
VF	CPR + defibrillation immediately + ALS protocol
Complete heart block	Atropine IV · transcutaneous pacing
Torsades de pointes	IV magnesium + stop QT-prolonging drugs
Hyperkalaemia	IV calcium + insulin-glucose

ABG — BAD First-Look · 5-Step Systematic · ROME

BAD — 5-Second Scan (do FIRST):
B=Breathing failure (PaO_2 <8 kPa) · A=Acidaemia (pH <7.2) · D=Dangerous CO_2 ($PaCO_2$ >6.5 + acidosis)
"First, I'll scan using BAD — no breathing failure, no severe acidaemia, no dangerous CO_2 retention."

Normal Ranges: pH 7.35–7.45 · $PaCO_2$ 4.7–6.0 kPa · HCO_3 22–26 mmol/L
5-Step Blueprint: pH (acid/alk?) → $PaCO_2$ (resp component) → HCO_3 (met component) → Primary disorder (ROME) → Compensation → A-a gradient

pH	$PaCO_2$	HCO_3	Primary Disorder	ROME
↓	↑	Normal/↑	Respiratory acidosis	Opposite
↓	Normal/↓	↓	Metabolic acidosis	Equal
↑	↓	Normal/↓	Respiratory alkalosis	Opposite
↑	Normal/↑	↑	Metabolic alkalosis	Equal

ROME Rule: Respiratory = Opposite (pH and CO_2 go in opposite directions). Metabolic = Equal (pH and HCO_3 go in same direction).
Winter's Formula (metabolic acidosis): Expected $PaCO_2 = (1.5 \times HCO_3) + 8 \pm 2$. If actual ≠ expected = mixed disorder.
A-a gradient wide: V/Q mismatch → PE, pneumonia, pulmonary oedema. Normal = hypoventilation/low FiO_2.

ABG Pattern Recognition · Emergency Actions

Scenario	ABG Pattern
Acute respiratory acidosis (opioid OD)	pH↓ · $PaCO_2$↑ · HCO_3 normal · A-a normal
COPD exacerbation (chronic resp acidosis)	pH↓/N · $PaCO_2$↑ · HCO_3↑ (compensation) · A-a normal
PE (respiratory alkalosis + type 1 RF)	pH↑ · $PaCO_2$↓ · PaO_2↓ · A-a wide
DKA / Sepsis (metabolic acidosis)	pH↓ · $PaCO_2$↓ · HCO_3↓ · high lactate/ketones
Vomiting/diuretics (metabolic alkalosis)	pH↑ · $PaCO_2$↑ · HCO_3↑
Salicylate OD (mixed)	Respiratory alkalosis + metabolic acidosis

ABG Emergency Actions:
PaO_2 <8 kPa → Oxygen (target 94–98%, 88–92% if COPD risk) · $PaCO_2$ >6.5 + acidosis → NIV/ventilation
pH <7.2 or >7.6 → Urgent ICU review · K+ >6.5 → IV calcium + insulin-glucose · K+ <2.5 → IV replacement + cardiac monitoring · Lactate ↑ → sepsis/shock/ischaemia

Clinical Correlation — ECG + ABG + Scenario

Scenario	ECG Finding	ABG Finding	Action
STEMI	ST elevation	Normal initially	Aspirin + immediate PCI
PE	Sinus tachy · S1Q3T3	Type 1 RF · wide A-a · resp alkalosis	O_2 + anticoagulation
COPD exacerbation	Tachy · P-pulmonale	Type 2 RF · resp acidosis	NIV + bronchodilators
DKA	Sinus tachycardia	Metabolic acidosis · low HCO_3	Fluids + insulin
Hyperkalaemia	Peaked T · wide QRS	Acidosis	IV calcium + insulin-glucose

Examiner Checklist

ECG ✓	ABG ✓
✓ KILL scan done first	✓ BAD scan done first
✓ Rate: correct method	✓ pH: acidaemia/alkalaemia
✓ Rhythm identified	✓ $PaCO_2$: respiratory component
✓ Axis: Lead I + aVF	✓ HCO_3: metabolic component
✓ PR/QRS/QTc assessed	✓ ROME applied — primary disorder
✓ LBBB + pain = STEMI equivalent	✓ Compensation assessed
✓ STEMI location (AIL)	✓ Winter's formula if met acidosis
✓ Special patterns checked	✓ A-a gradient assessed
✓ VT vs SVT distinction	✓ O_2 target stated (94-98%/88-92%)
✓ Emergency: immediate action	✓ Emergency: ICU escalation
✓ Clinical correlation	✓ Repeat ABG after intervention

Final Exam Mantra

ECG: KILL first → RRAIS systematic → AIL for STEMI locations → special patterns → act
RRAIS: Rate (300÷LgSq or 6s×10) · Rhythm · Axis (I+aVF) · Intervals · ST changes
ABG: BAD first → 5-step (pH→CO_2→HCO_3→ROME→compensation→A-a) → act
ROME: Respiratory=Opposite · Metabolic=Equal · Winter's for met acidosis
STEMI: immediate reperfusion · VT unstable: cardioversion · CHB: pacing · pH <7.2: ICU

Gold Closing — ECG:
"Systematically interpreted using RRAIS. Rate [X], rhythm [Y], axis [Z]. PR [normal/prolonged], QRS [narrow/wide], QTc [normal/prolonged]. ST [elevation/depression] in [leads]. Consistent with [diagnosis] — correlates with [symptoms]. Immediate management: [action]. Repeat ECG if symptoms persist. Escalate to cardiology/ICU."

Gold Closing — ABG:
"pH [acidaemia/alkalaemia]. $PaCO_2$ [high/low/normal] — [resp component]. HCO_3 [high/low/normal] — [met component]. Primary disorder: [resp/met acidosis/alkalosis]. Compensation [appropriate/mixed]. A-a [normal/wide]. Correlates with [clinical scenario]. Management: [oxygen/NIV/treat cause]. Repeat ABG after intervention."

KILL scan first 4 ECG emergencies	BAD scan first 4 ABG emergencies	RRAIS systematic rate rhythm axis intervals ST	ROME rule respiratory=opposite metabolic=equal	STEMI = AIL anterior inferior lateral
LBBB + pain STEMI equivalent	VT broad complex treat as VT if unsure	Winter's formula (1.5 x HCO3) + 8 +-2	A-a wide V/Q mismatch PE/pneumonia	Correlate always ECG/ABG to scenario

TOP 5 EXAMINER Q&A · ECG & ABG INTERPRETATION	
Q1. The ECG reading order that never fails?	Rate, rhythm, axis, intervals, then morphology by territory: P, PR, QRS, ST, T: and always: "old ECG for comparison".
Q2. The ST elevations that need the cath lab call?	Territorial ST elevation with reciprocal change: state the artery, then "activate primary PCI now".
Q3. The rhythm findings you must never miss?	VT, complete heart block, and a paced or pre-excited rhythm: each changes management immediately.
Q4. ABG in four steps?	Oxygenation, pH, respiratory component (CO2), metabolic component (bicarbonate/BE): then compensation and the anion gap.
Q5. The pattern of life-threatening asthma on ABG?	A normal or rising CO2 in an exhausted asthmatic: peri-arrest, not improvement.
CURVEBALL	The ECG is technically poor with artefact. Say it: "limited by artefact: I would repeat with attention to electrode contact": interpreting garbage confidently is the fail.

CHAPTER 71 · CHEST X-RAY & EMERGENCY IMAGING

RIPE · ABCDE · RAMP · CXR Pathologies · CT Head · Imaging Choice

CORE · CAUTION — INSTANT FAIL RISK · HIGH STAKES · A&E · Medical Take · Acute

Abbreviations used in this chapter: **DVT** Deep Vein Thrombosis · **PE** Pulmonary Embolism · **SAH** Subarachnoid Haemorrhage

THINK — Core: This is NOT a radiology test. It is a patient safety and decision-making test.
Fail Risk: Missing pneumothorax · Not escalating tension pneumothorax · Missing free air under diaphragm · Contrast without RAMP check

SAY — First 60 Seconds: "Check patient is stable. Interpret systematically. RIPE for image quality. ABCDE for findings. Look specifically for pneumothorax, mediastinal shift, free air."

RAMP (Before Contrast) · RIPE (Image Quality)

RAMP — Check Before ANY Contrast:
R=Renal (eGFR — avoid if eGFR <30) · A=Allergy (previous contrast reaction) · M=Metformin (withhold 48 hours before and after contrast if eGFR <30 — restart only after renal function confirmed stable) · P=Pregnancy (avoid if possible — prefer ultrasound)
Script: "Before contrast, I would check renal function, allergy history, metformin use, and pregnancy status."

	RIPE Check	Normal Finding	Script
R	Rotation	Spinous processes central	"Spinous processes central — no rotation."
I	Inspiration	≥6 anterior ribs	"Adequate inspiration — 6 anterior ribs."
P	Projection	PA vs AP noted	"PA view — heart size reliable."
E	Exposure	Vertebrae visible behind heart	"Vertebrae visible — good exposure."

ABCDE — Systematic CXR Interpretation

	Area	What to Check	Script
A	Airway & mediastinum	Trachea midline? Mediastinal width?	"Trachea midline, mediastinum normal."
B	Breathing & lungs	Lung fields symmetrical? Pneumothorax?	"Reviewing lung fields systematically."

	Area	What to Check	Script
C	Cardiac	CT ratio? Heart borders clear?	"CT ratio within normal limits."
D	Diaphragm	Costophrenic angles sharp? Free air?	"Costophrenic angles sharp."
E	Everything else	Bones, soft tissue, tubes, lines	"No abnormalities in bones or tubes."

Key Pathologies — Must-Not-Miss

Finding	Key Feature	Script
Pneumothorax	No peripheral lung markings + pleural edge	"Absent peripheral markings with visible pleural edge."
TENSION PNEUMOTHORAX	Mediastinal shift AWAY from side	"Tension pneumothorax — immediate decompression + senior NOW."
Pleural effusion	Blunted costophrenic angle, meniscus sign	"Blunting of costophrenic angle — pleural effusion."
Consolidation	Air bronchograms	"Airspace opacification with air bronchograms."
Collapse	Volume loss, shift TOWARDS	"Volume loss with shift towards — collapse."
Pulmonary oedema	Bilateral perihilar shadowing	"Perihilar opacification — pulmonary oedema."
Pneumoperitoneum	Free air UNDER diaphragm	"Free air under diaphragm — likely perforation — urgent surgical review."
Cardiomegaly	Enlarged cardiac shadow	"Enlarged cardiac silhouette — cardiomegaly."

Any life-threatening finding → escalate immediately to senior and initiate emergency management.
Normal CXR: "Does not exclude PE or early pneumonia — I will correlate clinically."

Consolidation vs Collapse vs Effusion

Feature	Consolidation	Collapse	Effusion
Air bronchograms	✓ Present	✗ Absent	✗ Absent
Volume loss	✗ No	✓ Yes	✗ No
Mediastinal shift	None	Towards collapse	Away if large

Feature	Consolidation	Collapse	Effusion
Costophrenic angle	Normal	Normal	CAUTION — Blunted

THINK — CT Head · Intracranial Bleeds · Imaging Choice

CT Head: Bright (hyperdense) = acute blood · Dark (hypodense) = ischaemia (may be normal early)
RED FLAG: Midline shift → urgent neurosurgical referral

Bleed Type	Shape	Key Feature
Extradural	Lens-shaped (biconvex)	Does NOT cross sutures
Subdural	Crescent-shaped	Crosses sutures
Subarachnoid (SAH)	Blood in sulci/cisterns	Diffuse, follows CSF spaces

Imaging Choice: CT = trauma/acute bleed/stroke (first) · MRI = spinal cord/soft tissue · Ultrasound = pregnancy/gallstones/DVT (avoid radiation)

Examiner Checklist

CXR Interpretation ✓	Safety + Escalation ✓
✓ Patient stability checked first	✓ Tension pneumothorax: immediate decompression
✓ RAMP before contrast	✓ Pneumoperitoneum: urgent surgical review
✓ RIPE image quality assessed	✓ CT head: midline shift = neurosurgical referral
✓ ABCDE systematic approach	✓ Clinical correlation stated
✓ Trachea midline noted	✓ Normal scan: does not exclude all conditions
✓ Key pathologies identified	✓ Comparison with previous imaging
✓ Consolidation vs collapse vs effusion	✓ Senior/radiology discussion mentioned
✓ CT head appearances known	✓ Documentation planned

Final Exam Mantra

RAMP before contrast: Renal · Allergy · Metformin · Pregnancy
RIPE image quality: Rotation · Inspiration · Projection · Exposure
ABCDE systematic: Airway · Breathing · Cardiac · Diaphragm · Everything else
Must-not-miss: Tension pneumothorax (shift AWAY) · Pneumoperitoneum · SAH · Midline shift
Consolidation = air bronchograms · Collapse = volume loss + shift towards · Effusion = blunted angle

Gold Closing:
"Patient stable. Image quality: RIPE — [adequate/suboptimal]. Systematic ABCDE: trachea [midline/deviated], lung fields [symmetrical/abnormal — describe], cardiac silhouette [normal/enlarged], costophrenic angles [sharp/blunted], bones/tubes [normal/abnormal]. Life-threatening findings: [none/describe]. Management: [escalate/action]. Clinical correlation: [link to presentation]."

RAMP first before any contrast	RIPE quality check before interpretation	ABCDE systematic every CXR always	Tension = shift AWAY immediate decompression	Free air = surgical pneumoperitoneum
Consolidation = AiBs air bronchograms	Collapse = shift TO volume loss towards	CT bright = blood dark = ischaemia	Extradural = lens subdural = crescent	Midline shift neurosurgical NOW

TOP 5 EXAMINER Q&A · CHEST X-RAY & EMERGENCY IMAGING	
Q1. The CXR system in one breath?	RIPE then ABCDE: Rotation, Inspiration, Projection, Exposure: then Airway, Breathing (lungs), Cardiac, Diaphragm, Everything else.
Q2. The findings that demand immediate action?	Tension features, large pneumothorax, white-out with mediastinal shift, free air under the diaphragm: name the emergency and the action.
Q3. How do you present an abnormal film?	Patient details and film quality first, the obvious abnormality described precisely, relevant negatives, then a clinical correlation.
Q4. Free air under the diaphragm means?	Perforated viscus until proven otherwise: nil by mouth, IV access, antibiotics, urgent surgical referral.
Q5. When do you say "CT"?	When the question is beyond the film: but state that an unstable patient is resuscitated first: the scanner is no place to arrest.
CURVEBALL	The film looks normal but the patient looks terrible. Say the sacred sentence: "a normal chest X-ray does not exclude PE, early pathology, or a clinical emergency: I treat the patient, not the film".

CHAPTER 72 · BLOOD TESTS & MULTI-DOMAIN CLINICAL REASONING

SCAN-60 · One-Story Integration · SBAR Escalation · Documentation

CORE · CAUTION — HIGH FAIL-RISK · HIGH STAKES

Abbreviations used in this chapter: AKI Acute Kidney Injury · NSAID Non-Steroidal Anti-Inflammatory Drug · PLAB Professional & Linguistic Assessments Board · STEMI ST-Elevation Myocardial Infarction

THINK — Core: This is NOT a knowledge test. It is a patient safety + decision-making test. Absolute Rule: Life-threatening abnormality → STOP → ACT immediately. Treat FIRST, think SECOND.

INSTANT FAIL: Not treating life-threat immediately · No ABCDE in unstable patient · Delay antibiotics (sepsis >1h) · No escalation · Silent interpretation · Rapid sodium correction

SAY — Golden Flow: SCAN → ACT → ABCDE (if unstable) → INTERPRET → LINK → ESCALATE

First 60 Seconds: "Check patient stable. Review results systematically — verbalising each value. Look for life-threatening abnormalities first. Act immediately if found. Then interpret and link to single diagnosis."

SCAN-60 — Danger Thresholds · Say Out Loud

See → STOP → ACT immediately. Do not continue interpretation until life-threat is addressed.

Test	**Danger Threshold**	**Immediate Action**
K^+	≥6.0 (or ≥5.5 + ECG changes)	Calcium gluconate → insulin/dextrose → ECG
Glucose	<3.0 mmol/L	IV glucose ± thiamine (if alcohol/malnourished)
Lactate	>2 concern / >4 ICU	>2 → consider sepsis (antibiotics within 1h) · >4 → ICU
Hb	<70 g/L	Crossmatch ± transfuse
Creatinine	↑>26 μmol/L or eGFR <30	AKI → IV fluids + stop nephrotoxins
Na^+	<120 / >155 mmol/L	Slow correction ONLY — NEVER correct rapidly

IF–THEN Action Core

Hyperkalaemia → Calcium gluconate FIRST (membrane stabilisation)
Hypoglycaemia → IV glucose immediately ± thiamine
Sepsis → Antibiotics within 1 hour
Severe anaemia → Transfuse if indicated · AKI → Stop nephrotoxins + IV fluids
Hyponatraemia → NEVER correct rapidly (osmotic demyelination)
Unstable patient → call for help → ABCDE immediately

ONE-STORY Multi-Domain Integration

Rule: Bloods + ECG + Imaging MUST tell ONE coherent story.
Structure: DATA → PATTERN → STORY → RISK
Script: "I will now integrate the blood results with ECG and imaging to form one clinical diagnosis."

Example	Findings	Examiner Gold Line
Acute STEMI	Troponin ↑ · ECG ST elevation · chest pain	"All findings fit — acute STEMI. Immediate reperfusion."
Sepsis + AKI	CRP ↑ · WCC ↑ · Creatinine ↑ · CXR consolidation	"This is sepsis complicated by AKI."
RED FLAG	Mild CRP · severe pain · normal imaging	"Findings don't match — escalate immediately."

SAY — SBAR Escalation · Documentation

SBAR Escalation — Escalate EARLY, before deterioration:
S=Situation: "Life-threatening abnormality — K^+ 6.4" · B=Background: "AKI, NSAID use"
A=Assessment: "Hyperkalaemia" · R=Recommendation: "Urgent senior review ± dialysis"

Documentation — Always Time-Stamp Actions:
Time reviewed · Critical value + time found · Treatment given · Working diagnosis · Escalation (SBAR at [time]) · Patient informed · Ongoing plan (repeat bloods in 2h + monitoring)
Patient communication: "This is serious — treating immediately. [X] means [simple explanation]. Involving specialist team. Call 999 if worse."

Examiner Checklist

SCAN-60 + Actions ✓	Integration + Communication ✓
✓ Patient stability checked first	✓ One-story integration stated
✓ SCAN-60 performed aloud	✓ SBAR escalation delivered early
✓ Life-threat identified immediately	✓ Antibiotics within 1h (sepsis)
✓ STOP → ACT before interpretation	✓ Patient explanation given simply

SCAN-60 + Actions ✓	**Integration + Communication ✓**
✓ ABCDE if unstable	✓ Documentation with timestamps
✓ K^+ ≥ 6.0: calcium gluconate first	✓ Hyponatraemia: slow correction only
✓ Lactate >4: ICU escalation	✓ Safety-net given
✓ AKI: stop nephrotoxins	✓ Repeat bloods planned

Final Exam Mantra

Scan → Spot danger → STOP → ACT → ABCDE → INTERPRET → ONE STORY → SBAR → Document → Speak

SCAN-60: K^+ ≥6.0 · Glucose <3.0 · Lactate >4 · Hb <70 · eGFR <30 · Na^+ <120/>155

If-Then: Hyperkalaemia=calcium gluconate · Hypoglycaemia=IV glucose · Sepsis=antibiotics <1h · Na^+=NEVER rapid

One Story: Bloods + ECG + imaging → single coherent diagnosis · Red flag: findings don't match = escalate

Gold Closing:

"SCAN-60 performed — identified [value/life-threat]. Treated immediately before interpretation. Results in context: [pattern]. One diagnosis: [X]. Escalated early (SBAR to [senior] at [time]). Patient explained. Safety-netted. Documented with timestamps. Repeat bloods in 2h + monitoring arranged."

SCAN-60 aloud verbalise every value	Life-threat = STOP ACT before interpreting	K+ ≥6.0 calcium gluconate first	Glucose <3.0 IV glucose ±thiamine	Lactate >4 ICU escalation now
Sepsis <1h ABx never delay antibiotics	Na+ slow only never rapid correction	One story rule bloods+ECG+imaging	SBAR early before deterioration	Timestamp always examiner checks this

Appendix 3A · OSCE TIMING MAPS

8-Minute Station Control Blueprint · Final 48 Hours Guide

History · Examination · Procedure · Prescribing · Data Interpretation · Joint Station

DISTINCTION — The 3 Things Examiners Really Mark:
Structure (organised?) · Safety (clinically safe?) · Sincerity (sound human and empathetic?)
Golden Rule: "You control the time. A calm 7:30 finish scores higher than a chaotic 8:00 rush."

Colour Phase Guide:
🟢 GREEN = Opening (rapport, consent, infection control) · 🟡 YELLOW = Data gathering (history/exam) · 🔵 BLUE = Assessment (synthesis + explanation) · 🟠 ORANGE = Closing (safety net + finish)
Final 60-Second Countdown: :60 Start summary · :45 Plan · :30 Ask questions · :15 Safety net · :05 Thank patient · :00 Exit calmly

HISTORY TAKING — 8-Minute Map

Time	Phase	Stage	Key Actions
0:00–0:30	GRN	ENTER & OPEN	Knock + smile · "Hello, I'm Dr ___" · Confirm name/DOB · Wash hands · "How can I help today?"
0:30–2:30	YEL	PRESENTING COMPLAINT	Open question first · SOCRATES (if pain) · Onset/duration/progression · 🔴 Empathy: "That sounds difficult."
2:30–4:00	YEL	FOCUSED REVIEW	Relevant systems review · Red flag symptoms · Severity assessment
4:00–5:00	YEL	BACKGROUND	PMH · Medications (incl. OTC) · Allergies (reaction + severity) · Family history
5:00–5:45	YEL	SOCIAL CONTEXT	Smoking/alcohol · Occupation · Living situation · Functional impact
5:45–6:30	BLU	ICE	Ideas · Concerns · Expectations
6:30–7:15	BLU	SUMMARY & PLAN	Structured summary · Working diagnosis · Initial plan · Investigations
7:15–8:00	ORG	CLOSE STRONGLY	Questions? · Clear safety net · Thank patient · Wash hands

EXAMINATION STATION — 8-Minute Map

Time	Phase	Stage	Key Actions
0:00–0:45	GRN	SET UP	Introduce · Confirm identity · Explain exam · Consent · Chaperone · Wash hands · Exposure + dignity · Position
0:45–1:15	YEL	GENERAL INSPECTION	End-of-bed assessment · Distress? · Around bed (O_2, IVs)
1:15–4:30	YEL	SYSTEMATIC EXAM	Structured sequence · Compare sides · Verbalise findings · Maintain patient comfort
4:30–5:15	YEL	SPECIAL TESTS	Relevant manoeuvres · Do not overdo
5:15–6:00	BLU	VERBALISE FINDINGS	"On examination I found..." · Summarise key positives/negatives
6:00–7:00	BLU	EXPLAIN & PLAN	Explain in plain language · Differentials · Next steps
7:00–8:00	ORG	CLOSE	Questions · Safety net · Re-cover patient · Wash hands · Thank & leave

PROCEDURE STATION — 8-Minute Map

Time	Phase	Stage	Key Actions
0:00–1:00	GRN	PRE-PROCEDURE	Introduce · Confirm identity · Explain · Allergies · Contraindications · Verbal consent · Chaperone
1:00–2:00	YEL	PREPARATION	Wash hands · Gather equipment · Position patient · Aseptic technique · Clean site
2:00–5:00	YEL	PERFORM PROCEDURE	Stepwise execution · Verbalise key steps · Communicate · Maintain sterility
5:00–6:00	BLU	AFTER PROCEDURE	Dispose sharps safely · Dress site · Label samples · Post-procedure checks
6:00–7:00	BLU	EXPLAIN AFTERCARE	What was done · What happens next · Possible complications
7:00–8:00	ORG	CLOSE	Questions · Safety net · Document verbally · Thank patient

PRESCRIBING STATION — 8-Minute Map

Time	Phase	Stage	Key Actions
0:00–0:30	GRN	ORIENT	Read scenario · Confirm age/weight · Check allergies
0:30–2:30	YEL	REVIEW	Current meds · Renal/liver function · Pregnancy status · Anticoagulation · Indication
2:30–6:00	BLU	WRITE PRESCRIPTION	Generic name · Dose (BNF) · Route · Frequency · Duration · Signature + printed name · Date + bleep
6:00–7:00	BLU	SAFETY CHECK	Interaction review · Dose adjustment · Allergy re-check · Monitoring needed
7:00–8:00	ORG	JUSTIFY	Explain indication · Dosing choice · Monitoring · Hand in confidently

DATA INTERPRETATION — 8-Minute Map

Time	Phase	Stage	Key Actions
0:00–1:00	GRN	ORIENT	Read task · Patient context · Demographics
1:00–3:00	YEL	SYSTEMATIC REVIEW	"I will interpret this systematically." · ECG: rate→rhythm→axis→intervals→ST · CXR: ABCDE · ABG: stepwise · Bloods: highlight abnormalities
3:00–4:00	YEL	SYNTHESISE	Link findings to presentation · Working diagnosis
4:00–6:00	BLU	MANAGEMENT	Immediate steps · Investigations · Referral/escalation
6:00–7:00	BLU	EXPLAIN (if required)	Plain language · Check understanding
7:00–8:00	ORG	CLOSE	Summary · Safety net · Documentation verbalised

JOINT STATION (History + Examination) — 8-Minute Map

Keep it tight. Do not over-collect data. Focused history + targeted examination only.

Time	Phase	Stage	Key Actions
0:00–0:30	GRN	OPEN	Introduce · Confirm identity · Wash hands
0:30–3:00	YEL	FOCUSED HISTORY	Key complaint only · Relevant PMH · Meds + allergies · ONE ICE question only

Time	Phase	Stage	Key Actions
3:00–5:30	YEL	FOCUSED EXAM	Targeted examination · Verbalise all findings
5:30–7:00	BLU	SYNTHESISE & EXPLAIN	Structured summary · Differentials · Management plan
7:00–8:00	ORG	CLOSE	Questions · Safety net · Thank patient

Universal Safety Net · If You Freeze

Universal Safety Net: "If you develop worsening pain, fever, shortness of breath, bleeding, confusion, or anything that worries you, please seek urgent medical help or attend A&E." Always adapt to scenario.

If You Freeze:
Pause. Breathe. Say: "Let me just gather my thoughts." Resume structure.
Silence feels longer to you than to the examiner.

DISTINCTION — Final Exam Morning Reminder

You do not need to be brilliant. You need to be:
Structured (organised?) · Safe (clinically safe?) · Kind (sound human and empathetic?)
If you look structured, safe, and sincere — you pass.

0:00-0:30 ENTER & OPEN	0:30-2:30 PRESENTING Cx	2:30-5:00 BACKGROUND + SOCIAL	5:45-6:30 ICE always	6:30-7:15 SUMMARY + PLAN
7:15-8:00 CLOSE + SAFETY NET	:60 to :00 Final countdown	Structure + Safe + Kind 3 examiner marks	Calm 7:30 finish beats chaotic 8:00	"Gather my thoughts" freeze recovery

Appendix 3B · PART 1 OF 2 · MOCK OSCE STATIONS 1–9

Chest Pain · Paediatric Fever · Breaking Bad News · Capacity · Drug Chart · Stroke · Anaphylaxis · Sepsis · Bronchiolitis

Candidate Brief · Layered Actor Script · Hidden Info · ☐ Marking Scheme · SAY — Debrief

STATION 1 — ACUTE CHEST PAIN (Possible ACS)

Candidate Brief:
55-year-old man, ED, sudden-onset central chest pain radiating to left arm, onset 45 minutes ago. Tasks: focused history · explain immediate management · outline investigations.

☐ Immediate Actions:

- ☐ ABC assessment — verbally acknowledge airway, breathing, circulation
- ☐ Attach monitoring: SpO_2, HR, BP, cardiac monitor
- ☐ ECG within 10 minutes — must state this explicitly
- ☐ Aspirin 300 mg orally — confirm no allergy first
- ☐ Oxygen ONLY if SpO_2 <94% — do NOT give routinely
- ☐ GTN sublingual if SBP >90 mmHg and pain unrelieved
- ☐ IV access + bloods: troponin, FBC, U&E, coag, glucose
- ☐ IV morphine + antiemetic for pain
- ☐ Escalate to cardiology/medical registrar immediately
- ☐ Calculate NEWS2

Layered Actor Script:

🟢 **DEFAULT:** Anxious but cooperative. Clutching chest. Diaphoretic.

🟡 **IF DELAY:** Wince and press chest harder. Breathe more shallowly. Grip arm.

🔴 **IF NO ESCALATION:** "Doctor, I feel dizzy now and my arm is completely numb."

SAY — ACTOR PROMPT: "Doctor, the pain is getting worse and going up into my jaw now."

Hidden Info — reveal only if candidate asks directly:

Jaw/neck radiation: Yes — to left arm and jaw
Previous episodes: Similar episode 3 weeks ago, self-resolved — did not seek help
Family history: Father had heart attack at 58
Medications: Amlodipine for blood pressure — missed last 2 doses
Allergies: NKDA

Domain (marks)	Criteria
Communication (4)	Introduces + confirms ID · Clear reassuring language · Acknowledges pain/distress · Checks understanding

Domain (marks)	Criteria
Clinical Assessment (6)	Characterises pain (SOCRATES) · Risk factors · Associated symptoms · Haemodynamic status · ECG within 10 min · Recognises ACS
Management (6)	Aspirin 300mg (allergy check) · O_2 only if <94% · GTN/opioid · Bloods incl troponin · Cardiology escalation · Monitoring + repeat ECG plan
Safety (4)	Time-critical emergency · Senior escalation · Calm composure · Patient not left alone

Critical Fail Triggers:

✗ Routine oxygen without checking SpO_2

✗ ECG delayed beyond 10 minutes or not requested

✗ Fails to escalate to cardiology/senior

✗ Misses aspirin or gives without allergy check

✗ Ignores ABC — begins history without patient assessment

SAY — Examiner Debrief Prompts:

- ECG shows ST elevation II, III, aVF. Diagnosis and next 60 seconds?
- Why did you withhold oxygen? When would you give it?
- Troponin returns at 650 ng/L. Does that change your plan?
- His wife is in the waiting room. How do you communicate the diagnosis?

NOTE — Memory Anchor: AMEN → ABC + Monitor + ECG within 10 min + eNquire → Aspirin + Escalate + NEWS2

STATION 2 — PAEDIATRIC FEVER & BREATHING DIFFICULTY

Candidate Brief:

2-year-old boy, ED, fever 24 hours, breathing faster than usual. Tasks: history from parent · assess severity · immediate management plan.

☐ **Immediate Actions:**

☐ ABC — respiratory rate, effort, SpO_2, skin colour

☐ Oxygen if SpO_2 <92% via face mask or nasal cannula

☐ Assess work of breathing: nasal flaring, intercostal recession, grunting

☐ Assess hydration: skin turgor, capillary refill, urine output

☐ Temperature + Paediatric Early Warning Score (PEWS)

☐ ASK EXPLICITLY about non-blanching rash — meningococcal risk

☐ Escalate to paediatric team if any red flag present

☐ IV/IM access if moderate-severe dehydration or respiratory compromise

Layered Actor Script:

🟢 **DEFAULT:** Worried but calm parent. Child visibly fussy, pulling at ears, flushed.

🟡 **IF DELAY:** "He's breathing so fast — is that normal?" Look increasingly anxious.

🔴 **IF NO ESCALATION:** "I think he's getting worse — look at his tummy moving when he breathes."

SAY — ACTOR PROMPT: "Doctor, my child is breathing very fast and his lips look a bit bluish."

Hidden Info — reveal only if candidate asks directly:

Feeding: Refused two feeds today — only small amounts of fluid taken

Urine output: Fewer wet nappies — only 2 in last 24 hours (normal 6+)

Immunisations: Up to date — had MMR 2 weeks ago

Rash: No rash noted — if non-blanching asked specifically: "I'm not sure, I haven't checked"

Fever height: Temperature 39.4°C at home (paracetamol given 2 hours ago)

Domain (marks)	Criteria
Communication (4)	Introduces, addresses parent by name · Reassures honestly · Jargon-free · Checks understanding
Clinical Assessment (6)	Fever: onset/duration/height/antipyretics · Breathing: rate/effort/SpO_2 · Feeding/nappies · Red flags: rash/seizure/cyanosis · Immunisations + contacts · General appearance
Management (6)	O_2 if SpO_2 <92% · Antipyretics · Fluid assessment/IV if dehydrated · Paediatric review · Safety-net advice · Follow-up with timeframe
Safety (4)	Recognises respiratory distress · Escalates when red flag present · No discharge without safety net · Child-centred throughout

Critical Fail Triggers:

✗ Fails to assess SpO_2 or work of breathing early

✗ Discharges or plans discharge without safety-net advice

✗ Misses reduced urine output/dehydration when enquired about

✗ Fails to enquire about non-blanching rash

SAY — Examiner Debrief Prompts:

- SpO_2 drops to 89% while you are talking. Next 30 seconds?
- Mother asks: is this meningitis? How do you respond?
- PEWS score is 6. What does this trigger?
- Why did you ask specifically about urine output and wet nappies?

NOTE — Memory Anchor: SAFE-D → SpO_2 + Assess WOB + Fever history + Escalate + Dehydration check + DON'T FORGET RASH

SAY — STATION 3 — BREAKING BAD NEWS (SPIKES + NURSE)

Candidate Brief:
Mrs Ahmed, 47, biopsy confirms invasive ductal carcinoma. Tasks: explain results using SPIKES · respond to emotion using NURSE · outline next steps.

☐ **Immediate Actions:**
- ☐ Confirm private setting, tissues available, enough time allocated
- ☐ Establish what patient already knows — Perception step
- ☐ Ask how much information she wants — Invitation step
- ☐ Deliver warning shot before giving diagnosis
- ☐ Use the word "cancer" clearly — do not use euphemisms
- ☐ Allow silence after delivering news — do not fill it
- ☐ Respond to emotion using NURSE before any further clinical information
- ☐ Outline next steps: MDT, oncology referral, CNS nurse, written information
- ☐ Offer follow-up appointment and direct contact number
- ☐ Document the conversation accurately

Layered Actor Script:
🟢 **DEFAULT:** Calm, slightly anxious. Brought a notepad. Expects good news.
🟡 **IF DELAY:** Silently stunned. Long pause. Eyes fill with tears. Does not speak.
🔴 **IF NO ESCALATION:** "I'm sorry, I just need a moment." Begins to cry.
SAY — ACTOR PROMPT: "Am I going to die? / How long have I got? / What about my children — they're only 8 and 11."

Hidden Info — reveal only if candidate asks directly:
What she knows: Googled breast lump — suspects cancer but hasn't told family
Support at home: Husband works abroad. Two children aged 8 and 11
Information preferences: Wants to be told everything directly — no softening
Occupation: She is a nurse — understands medical terminology if used carefully
Previous biopsies: One previous benign lump removed age 39

Domain (marks)	Criteria
Communication (10)	Private setting · Warning shot · Perception first · Invitation · Says "cancer" clearly · Pauses after delivery · NURSE response · Does not continue while distressed · CNS/support offered · Summarises plan
Clinical Content (5)	Explains invasive ductal carcinoma · MDT required · Treatment pathways · Oncology referral · Cancer support helpline + leaflet
Professionalism (5)	Maintains warmth · Respects dignity · No unsolicited prognosis statistics · Adapts to nurse · Clear follow-up + written summary

Critical Fail Triggers:

✗ Delivers diagnosis without warning shot

✗ Continues talking while patient is crying or distressed

✗ Uses euphemisms only — never says "cancer" clearly

✗ Volunteers detailed prognosis statistics unprompted

✗ Fails to offer specialist referral or next steps

SAY — Examiner Debrief Prompts:

- "How long have I got?" — how did you handle that, and why?
- Why did you pause after delivering the diagnosis?
- She told you she is a nurse — did that change your approach?
- What would you document after this consultation, and who would you inform?

NOTE — Memory Anchor: SPIKES+NURSE → Setting → Perception → Invitation → Knowledge → Empathy (NURSE) → Strategy

STATION 4 — CAPACITY ASSESSMENT (Refusing Insulin)

Candidate Brief:

Mr Jones, 78, T1DM, refusing insulin. BG 24 mmol/L. Tasks: formal MCA 2005 capacity assessment · explore reasons · document and formulate plan.

☐ **Immediate Actions:**

☐ Introduce and establish rapport BEFORE any assessment

☐ Stage 1: Confirm impairment or disturbance of mind or brain

☐ Understand: Can he explain what insulin does and consequences of refusal?

☐ Retain: Can he recall explanation given moments earlier?

☐ Weigh: Can he use information to make a decision (even unwise)?

☐ Communicate: Can he state his decision clearly?

☐ Explore reasons for refusal — open questions, do not judge

☐ Explain DKA risk in plain language — check understanding

☐ Offer alternatives: reduced dose, very close monitoring

☐ Document findings: capacity present or absent + reasons

☐ Escalate to senior if capacity lacking or situation unclear

Layered Actor Script:

🟢 **DEFAULT:** Polite but firm. Arms folded. Not hostile — just certain.

🟡 **IF DELAY:** "I've had diabetes for 40 years. I know when I need insulin and when I don't."

🔴 **IF NO ESCALATION:** "I'd like you to leave please. I haven't agreed to anything."

SAY — ACTOR PROMPT: "I'm not having it. And that's my final word on the matter."

Hidden Info — reveal only if candidate asks directly:
Why refusing insulin: Bad hypo last month — found collapsed. Terrified of insulin.
Understanding of risk: Knows high sugar can damage kidneys and eyes
What he thinks: Can manage with diet — has done it before
Support at home: Lives alone since wife died 18 months ago
Advance Decision: No written advance decision in place

Domain (marks)	Criteria
Communication (4)	Introduces first · Non-judgemental open questions · Explains findings clearly · Respects dignity
Capacity Assessment (8)	Stage 1 impairment · Understand · Retain · Weigh · Communicate · Explores refusal reason (hypo fear) · Documents conclusion · Unwise ≠ incapacity
Management (4)	Explains DKA risk (glucose 24, coma/death) · Offers alternatives · Documents refusal if capacity present · Best interests + senior if capacity absent
Safety (4)	No coercion · Fully documented · Senior escalated if absent · Duty + autonomy balanced

Critical Fail Triggers:
- ✗ Administers insulin without completing capacity assessment
- ✗ Uses coercion, threats or emotional manipulation
- ✗ Fails to explore reason for refusal — misses hypoglycaemia fear
- ✗ Does not document findings or escalate when capacity is absent

SAY — Examiner Debrief Prompts:
- He has capacity and refuses. What do you do now — step by step?
- He cannot explain DKA. Does that alone mean he lacks capacity?
- His daughter arrives and demands you give the insulin. What do you say?
- What is the difference between an unwise decision and incapacity?

NOTE — Memory Anchor: URWC → Understand + Retain + Weigh + Communicate → Document + Escalate if absent

STATION 5 — INPATIENT DRUG CHART (CAP, Penicillin Allergy)

Candidate Brief:
Mr Brown, 62, CAP, CURB-65 = 2, penicillin allergic, creatinine 140 μmol/L. Tasks: allergy history · prescribe correctly · explain choice.

☐ **Immediate Actions:**

☐ Ask about allergy FIRST — before touching drug chart

☐ Characterise reaction: rash vs anaphylaxis, timing, severity

☐ Confirm indication: CAP with CURB-65 score 2

☐ Correct agent: Doxycycline 200mg day 1 then 100mg OD, or Clarithromycin 500mg BD

☐ Check renal function: creatinine 140 — review renally-cleared drugs

☐ Document allergy in red on drug chart with reaction type

☐ Correct dose, route (oral if tolerating), frequency, duration (5 days)

☐ Sign and date with GMC number and bleep

☐ Explain choice to patient: why not penicillin, what chosen, what to watch for

Layered Actor Script:

🟢 **DEFAULT:** Cooperative, coughing, short of breath. Concerned about allergies.

🟡 **IF DELAY:** Waits until pen on chart then: "Doctor — aren't you going to check my allergies first?"

🔴 **IF NO ESCALATION:** "Is that not penicillin? I thought I told the nurse I'm allergic."

SAY — ACTOR PROMPT: "Last time I had penicillin I came out in a rash all over my back. I hope whatever you give me is safe."

Hidden Info — reveal only if candidate asks directly:

Allergy reaction type: Rash only — no anaphylaxis, no airway compromise

Timing of reaction: After about 5 days of a course, 3 years ago

Other allergies: NKDA to other drugs

Current medications: Bisoprolol 5mg OD · Ramipril 5mg OD · Atorvastatin 40mg nocte

Renal function: Creatinine 140 = mild-moderate impairment. Dose check required.

Domain (marks)	Criteria
Communication (4)	Introduces + confirms ID · Allergy asked first · Explains choice in plain language · Checks understanding
Prescribing Safety (8)	Allergy reaction type (rash vs anaphylaxis) · Documents allergy in red · Correct agent (doxy/clarith, not penicillin) · Correct dose · Correct route · 5 days duration · Signed + dated · Renal function reviewed
Clinical Reasoning (4)	Why penicillin avoided · CURB-65 = 2 significance · IV route if deteriorating · 48h review plan
Safety (4)	No prescription without allergy check · Explains duration to patient · Plans monitoring · Escalates if reaction

Critical Fail Triggers:

✗ Prescribes penicillin/amoxicillin despite documented allergy

✗ Fails to ask about allergy before prescribing

✗ Does not characterise reaction type (rash vs anaphylaxis)

✗ INCORRECT DURATION — CAP = 5 days, NOT 7

✗ Omits dose, frequency, duration, or signature from chart

SAY — Examiner Debrief Prompts:

- Why does reaction type — rash vs anaphylaxis — matter for your prescribing decision?
- What is CURB-65 and why does a score of 2 change management?
- Creatinine is 140. Which antibiotic classes need dose adjustment and why?
- He develops a new widespread rash 6 hours later. What do you do?

NOTE — Memory Anchor: DDRF-AR+5DAYS → Drug + Dose (renal check) + Route + Freq + Allergy (reaction type) + Review + Duration (5 days)

THINK — STATION 6 — ACUTE STROKE (Time-Critical Thrombolysis)

Candidate Brief:

Mr Khan, 67, right arm weakness and slurred speech, onset ~3 hours ago. HTN + AF.
Tasks: rapid clinical assessment · time-critical management · communicate and escalate.

☐ **Immediate Actions:**

☐ FAST: Face, Arms, Speech, Time — document time of onset
☐ ABC — ensure airway, IV access
☐ Check blood glucose immediately — hypoglycaemia mimics stroke
☐ BP + cardiac monitoring — check for AF on rhythm strip
☐ Urgent CT head (non-contrast) BEFORE thrombolysis
☐ Call stroke team IMMEDIATELY — time is brain
☐ Check INR urgently — patient on warfarin
☐ Do NOT give aspirin until CT confirms no haemorrhage
☐ Document NIHSS score or equivalent deficit assessment
☐ If ischaemic + within 4.5h window: discuss thrombolysis with stroke team
☐ Check thrombolysis contraindications: warfarin/INR, recent surgery, bleeding

Layered Actor Script:

🟢 **DEFAULT:** Confused, frightened. Slurred speech. Right arm hanging. Wife at bedside.
🟡 **IF DELAY:** "Doctor, his face looks funny on one side — is that normal?" (Wife)
🔴 **IF NO ESCALATION:** "Doctor, he's trying to speak but he can't get the words out. Please help him."
SAY — ACTOR PROMPT: "He was fine this morning. We were having breakfast and then he just... dropped his cup."

Hidden Info — reveal only if candidate asks directly:
Exact time of onset: Confirmed 3 hours ago — within 4.5-hour thrombolysis window
Medications: Warfarin for AF · amlodipine for BP
Contraindications: No recent surgery, no active bleeding, no prior stroke in 3 months
Blood glucose: BM is 5.4 mmol/L if candidate checks
BP on arrival: 184/96 mmHg

Domain (marks)	Criteria
Communication (4)	Introduces to patient + wife · Explains clearly · Simple language (patient dysphasia) · Conveys urgency without panic

Domain (marks)	Criteria
Clinical Assessment (6)	FAST + time of onset · Blood glucose (mimic exclusion) · BP/HR/AF · Focal deficit · 3-hour window established · Contraindications enquired
Management (6)	Stroke team called immediately · Urgent non-contrast CT · INR checked · No aspirin until CT · Thrombolysis if ischaemic + window + INR ≤1.7 · Post-CT plan (aspirin, statin, swallow, DVT)
Safety (4)	No delay in escalation · No aspirin before CT · Documents time/FAST/BP/glucose · Communicates urgency professionally

Critical Fail Triggers:

✗ Fails to perform FAST or document time of onset

✗ Gives aspirin BEFORE CT excludes haemorrhage

✗ Delays calling stroke team for further junior assessment

✗ Fails to check blood glucose — misses hypoglycaemia mimic

✗ Fails to check INR in patient on warfarin

SAY — Examiner Debrief Prompts:

- CT: no haemorrhage. Onset 3 hours. INR 1.2. What do you do next exactly?
- INR comes back 2.8. Does this change your thrombolysis plan?
- What is the 4.5-hour window and why does it matter?
- Wife asks: will he be able to speak again? How do you answer?

NOTE — Memory Anchor: FAST-CT → Face+Arms+Speech+Time → Glucose → BP+Monitor → CT head → Stroke team → Thrombolysis window → Check INR

STATION 7 — ANAPHYLAXIS (RCUK Algorithm)

Candidate Brief:

Ms Patel, 28, collapsed in clinic waiting room after lunch. Conscious but respiratory distress + generalised urticaria. Tasks: recognise anaphylaxis · RCUK algorithm · communicate and escalate.

☐ **Immediate Actions:**

☐ Remove trigger if identifiable — call for help simultaneously

☐ ABC — position: sit up if breathless, lie flat + legs elevated if shocked

☐ IM adrenaline 0.5mg (0.5mL of 1:1000) into anterolateral thigh IMMEDIATELY

☐ High-flow oxygen via non-rebreather mask

☐ IV access — give 500–1000mL crystalloid if hypotensive

☐ Repeat IM adrenaline after 5 minutes if no improvement

☐ If no response after 2 IM doses → refractory anaphylaxis: IV adrenaline infusion + further IV fluids (senior/ICU-led). Routine antihistamines/steroids NOT recommended (RCUK 2021); non-sedating oral antihistamine only after stabilisation for skin symptoms

☐ Cardiac monitoring — ECG leads + SpO_2

☐ Call 999/crash team/ICU — escalate immediately

☐ Observe minimum 6–12 hours post-reaction for biphasic response

☐ Prescribe adrenaline auto-injector on discharge + refer to allergy clinic

Layered Actor Script:

🟢 **DEFAULT:** Distressed, wheezing audible. Flushed, swollen lips. Scratching arms.

🟡 **IF DELAY:** "I can't breathe properly... it's getting tighter."

🔴 **IF NO ESCALATION:** Stridor develops. Actor holds throat. Conveys panic non-verbally.

SAY — ACTOR PROMPT: "I feel really strange... my throat is swelling up. I had a chicken wrap from downstairs."

Hidden Info — reveal only if candidate asks directly:

Trigger: Peanuts — sesame paste in the wrap. Must ask about contents.

Previous reactions: One previous mild reaction to nuts aged 16 — never treated

Epipen: No — never been prescribed one

Medications: OCP only. NKDA to medications.

Pregnancy: Not pregnant. (Pregnancy is NOT a contraindication to adrenaline — never delay treatment.)

Domain (marks)	Criteria
Communication (4)	Calm self-identification · Clear instructions to bystanders · Explains to patient · Documents time + treatment
Recognition (4)	Urticaria + wheeze + stridor + collapse after allergen · Identifies trigger (peanut/sesame) · Assesses airway compromise · Assesses circulatory status
Management (8)	IM adrenaline 0.5mg 1:1000 anterolateral thigh immediately · Correct position · High-flow O_2 · IV access + crystalloid · Repeat at 5 min · Refractory (no response ×2) → IV adrenaline infusion + fluids · No routine antihistamine/steroid (RCUK 2021) · ICU escalation · 6–12h observation
Safety (4)	No delay — adrenaline first · Correct concentration: 1:1000 (not 1:10,000) · Escalates immediately · Allergy clinic + auto-injector planned

Critical Fail Triggers:

✗ Delays adrenaline or substitutes it with an antihistamine/steroid (adrenaline is the only first-line drug)

✗ Uses wrong concentration: 1:10,000 IM (cardiac arrest dose)

✗ Gives adrenaline IV instead of IM without ICU monitoring

✗ Fails to escalate — attempts to manage alone in clinic

SAY — Examiner Debrief Prompts:

- Why is the anterolateral thigh the preferred injection site?
- She improves then deteriorates 30 minutes later. What is this called and what do you do?
- Difference between 1:1000 and 1:10,000 adrenaline and when each is used?
- Before discharging her, what must you arrange?

NOTE — Memory Anchor: AIR → Adrenaline IM 0.5mg 1:1000 → In anterolateral thigh → Repeat at 5 min → O_2 + Fluids + Escalate

STATION 8 — SEPSIS (Sepsis-6 within 1 Hour)

Candidate Brief:

Mrs White, 71, confusion and rigors, urinary catheter in situ. HR 118, BP 88/52, RR 28, Temp 38.9°C, SpO_2 94%. NEWS2 = 10. Tasks: Sepsis-6 bundle · immediate management · communicate and escalate.

☐ **Immediate Actions:**

☐ TAKE: Blood cultures ×2 from two sites BEFORE antibiotics
☐ TAKE: Lactate/VBG — target <2 mmol/L
☐ TAKE: Urine output measurement — hourly catheter monitoring
☐ GIVE: IV broad-spectrum antibiotics within 1 hour of recognition
☐ GIVE: IV crystalloid 500mL bolus if lactate >2 or MAP <65
☐ GIVE: Oxygen — target SpO_2 >94%
☐ Escalate to senior/ICU if lactate >4, not improving after fluids
☐ Review catheter — still indicated? Source control.
☐ Calculate NEWS2 + document time of recognition (NOT admission time)

Layered Actor Script:

🟢 **DEFAULT:** Confused but rousable. Shivering. Very pale. Barely responds.

🟡 **IF DELAY:** Groans. BP drops further. Nurse: "Her pressure is dropping, doctor."

🔴 **IF NO ESCALATION:** "She's not responding to me properly now." Nurse looks frightened.

SAY — ACTOR PROMPT: "Doctor... I feel so cold... I can't stop shaking. Something is very wrong."

Hidden Info — reveal only if candidate asks directly:

Source: Catheter-associated UTI — catheter in situ 8 days
Lactate: Lactate 4.2 mmol/L — reveals if candidate orders VBG/lactate
Urine output: Only 15mL in last 2 hours
Allergies: No known drug allergies
Last blood cultures: None taken yet today

Domain (marks)	**Criteria**
Communication (4)	Clear calm introduction · Explains to confused patient · SBAR to nursing team · SBAR escalation to senior
Recognition (4)	Sepsis: infection + organ dysfunction + haemodynamic compromise · Source: catheter UTI · NEWS2 · Lactate 4.2 = severe
Sepsis-6 (8)	Blood cultures before antibiotics · Lactate ordered · Urine output monitoring · IV ABx within 1h · 500mL crystalloid · O_2 for SpO_2 >94% · Source control (catheter) · ICU escalated (lactate 4.2)
Safety (4)	No ABx delay · Escalates immediately (severity) · Documents time zero · Recognises septic shock

Critical Fail Triggers:

X Gives antibiotics before blood cultures without acknowledging sequence

X Fails to give IV fluids despite BP 88/52

X Does not escalate to senior/ICU despite lactate 4.2

X Misses urine output monitoring as Sepsis-6 element

SAY — Examiner Debrief Prompts:

- Lactate 4.2 mmol/L. What does this mean and what does it trigger?
- Why must blood cultures be taken BEFORE antibiotics?
- After 2 hours BP still 82/50 despite 1.5L fluid. What next?
- How do you escalate this to ICU using SBAR?

NOTE — Memory Anchor: Sepsis-6 → Cultures + Lactate + Urine (TAKE) → Antibiotics + Fluids + O_2 (GIVE) → Escalate + Document TIME ZERO (recognition, NOT admission)

STATION 9 — PAEDIATRIC BRONCHIOLITIS (NICE NG9)

Candidate Brief:

6-week-old girl, 3-day history of runny nose, cough, difficulty feeding, wheeze. Tasks: history from parents · assess severity · NICE NG9 management.

☐ **Immediate Actions:**

☐ ABC — RR, SpO_2, work of breathing, colour, tone

☐ Oxygen via nasal cannula if SpO_2 <92%

☐ Assess severity: mild (SpO_2 >95%, feeding >75%) / moderate / severe

☐ Establish feeding history: volume, time per feed, fatiguing

☐ Consider NG tube feeding if taking <50–75% of normal volume

☐ IV fluids if inadequate oral/NG or RR too high for safe feeding

☐ Do NOT perform routine nasal suctioning (NICE NG9)

☐ Do NOT prescribe bronchodilators, steroids, or antibiotics unless secondary infection

☐ Escalate to paediatric senior: premature infant + apnoea episode

☐ Admit for monitoring: SpO_2, RR, feeding volumes

Layered Actor Script:

🟢 **DEFAULT:** Both parents present. Mother anxious, father quiet. Baby tachypnoeic.

🟡 **IF DELAY:** "She keeps going a bluey colour around the mouth when she cries. Is that serious?"

🔴 **IF NO ESCALATION:** "This is our first baby. We've never seen her like this. Please do something."

SAY — ACTOR PROMPT: "She won't feed properly. She starts and then pulls away. And her breathing sounds so noisy."

Hidden Info — reveal only if candidate asks directly:
Feeding: Taking only 30% of normal feed volume over last 24 hours — fatiguing
Apnoea: One episode at home — "she went quiet and stopped breathing for a few seconds"
Gestation: Born at 34 weeks — premature, higher risk of severe bronchiolitis
RSV exposure: Older sibling (age 3) has had a cold for one week
SpO_2: Currently 91% on air (moderate severity)

Domain (marks)	Criteria
Communication (4)	Introduces, addresses both parents · Jargon-free · Explains bronchiolitis · Honest + reassuring about admission
Clinical Assessment (6)	3-day progression · Feeding <30% (hidden key finding) · Apnoea at home (critical) · SpO_2 91% (moderate) · Prematurity: 34 weeks · Respiratory: RR/flaring/recession/grunting
Management (6)	O_2 via nasal cannula (SpO_2 ≥94%) · NG feeding (<50% volume, fatiguing) · Admits for monitoring · No routine suctioning (NICE NG9) · No bronchodilators/steroids/ABx · Paediatric senior escalation (premature + apnoea + SpO_2 91%)
Safety (4)	Apnoea = high-risk escalation · Prematurity recognised · No guideline-contraindicated treatments · Safety-net before discharge discussion

Critical Fail Triggers:

✗ Performs routine nasopharyngeal suctioning — contradicts NICE NG9
✗ Prescribes salbutamol, steroids or antibiotics without indication
✗ Fails to identify apnoea episode when asked directly
✗ Discharges without monitoring plan given SpO_2 91% and feeding difficulties

SAY — Examiner Debrief Prompts:

- Why does NICE NG9 advise against routine suctioning? What changed?
- Born at 34 weeks. Why does prematurity change your risk assessment?
- Father asks: should she have salbutamol like his nephew? What do you say?
- At what SpO_2 threshold would you escalate to CPAP or intubation?

NOTE — Memory Anchor: SAFE-B → SpO_2 + Assess severity + Feed history + Escalate (premature+apnoea) + Supportive (NO suctioning, NO bronchodilators, NO steroids)

Part 1 Rapid Reference — Stations 1–9

Stn	Station	Memory Anchor	Key Hidden Info	Critical Fail
1	Chest Pain	AMEN: ABC+Monitor+ECG+eNquire+Aspirin+Escalate	Jaw radiation / missed antihypertensives	Routine O_2 without SpO_2 · delay ECG

Stn	Station	Memory Anchor	Key Hidden Info	Critical Fail
2	Paeds Fever	SAFE-D: SpO_2+WOB+Fever+Escalate+Dehydration	Urine output reduced / rash not checked	No safety-net · miss rash question
3	Bad News	SPIKES+NURSE: Setting→Perception→Invite→Knowledge→Empathy→Strategy	Patient is nurse · husband abroad · children 8+11	No warning shot · never says "cancer"
4	Capacity	URWC: Understand+Retain+Weigh+Communicate→Document	Refuses due to hypoglycaemia fear (last month)	Treat without assessing · coerce patient
5	Drug Chart	DDRF-AR+5DAYS: Drug+Dose(renal)+Route+Freq+Allergy+Review	Reaction = rash only · creatinine 140	Prescribe penicillin · WRONG duration (5 not 7)
6	Stroke	FAST-CT+INR: FAST+Glucose+CT+Stroke team+Thrombolysis	Onset 3h ago · on warfarin · INR not checked	No CT before aspirin · delay stroke team · miss INR
7	Anaphylaxis	AIR: Adrenaline IM 1:1000→anterolateral thigh→Repeat+O_2+Fluids	Peanuts in wrap · no Epipen ever prescribed	Antihistamine first · wrong concentration (1:10,000)
8	Sepsis	Sepsis-6+TIME ZERO: Cultures+Lactate+Urine→ABx+Fluids+O_2	Lactate 4.2 · catheter 8 days · urine 15mL/2h	ABx before cultures · miss TIME ZERO documentation
9	Bronchiolitis	SAFE-B: SpO_2+Assess+Feed+Escalate+Supportive(no suction)	Apnoea at home · born 34 weeks · SpO_2 91%	Routine suctioning · prescribe salbutamol/steroids

Part 2 (Stations 10–18): PPH · Reduced FM · Self-Harm · Alcohol Withdrawal · Consent · Insulin · ECG Interpretation · Telephone Consultation · Angry Relative

Appendix 3C · PART 2 OF 2 · MOCK OSCE STATIONS 10–18

PPH · Reduced FM · Self-Harm · Alcohol Withdrawal · Consent · Insulin · ECG/Hyperkalaemia · Telephone · Angry Relative

Candidate Brief · Layered Actor · Hidden Info · ☐ Marking Scheme · SAY — Debrief

STATION 10 — POSTPARTUM HAEMORRHAGE (PPH)

Candidate Brief:

Mrs Green, 28, SVD, ongoing heavy vaginal bleeding ~900mL (now >1100mL). Placenta delivered 5 min ago. Uterus boggy. Tasks: recognise and manage PPH · emergency team response · communicate and escalate.

☐ Immediate Actions:

☐ CALL FOR HELP immediately: senior obstetrician, anaesthetist, midwife

☐ ABC — airway, RR, SpO_2, HR, BP

☐ Two large-bore IV cannulae (14–16G) — both antecubital fossae

☐ Bloods: FBC, clotting, crossmatch 4 units, group & save, U&E — URGENT

☐ IV crystalloid bolus 500–1000mL while awaiting blood products

☐ Catheterise bladder — full bladder impairs uterine contraction

☐ Uterine massage / bimanual compression

☐ Uterotonics: Oxytocin 40 IU infusion (FIRST LINE), ergometrine if no HT, misoprostol 1000mcg PR

☐ Activate Major Haemorrhage Protocol if EBL >1500mL or haemodynamically unstable

☐ Document: time, EBL, drugs, BP, HR, interventions

Layered Actor Script:

🟢 **DEFAULT:** Conscious but pale. Frightened. Holding baby. Partner present.

🟡 **IF DELAY:** "Doctor, the bleeding is not slowing down. Should someone else be here?"

🔴 **IF NO ESCALATION:** "She's gone very pale and feels faint now." (Midwife urgently)

SAY — ACTOR PROMPT: "Is my baby OK? What's happening to me? I feel very dizzy."

Hidden Info — reveal only if asked directly:

Estimated blood loss: Total now 1100mL and ongoing — if asked midwife

Placenta: Delivered intact — no retained products suspected

Tone: Uterus is soft and boggy (uterine atony = primary cause)

Oxytocin given: 10 IU given in third stage — has not resolved bleeding

Bladder: Catheter not yet in — if asked, midwife will insert

Group and save: Not yet sent — no crossmatch yet

Domain (marks)	Criteria
Communication (4)	Introduces + reassures patient/partner · Explains clearly · Clear team instructions · Updates at each step

Domain (marks)	Criteria
Recognition & Resuscitation (6)	Recognises PPH (EBL >500mL) · Calls senior + anaesthetist · Two large-bore cannulae · IV fluids · FBC/clotting/crossmatch/G&S · Oxygen
Uterotonic Management (6)	Identifies uterine atony (boggy uterus) · Catheterises bladder · Uterine massage/compression · Oxytocin 40 IU infusion · Second-line: ergometrine/misoprostol · Major Haemorrhage Protocol when threshold reached
Safety (4)	Does not leave patient for equipment · Escalates early · Continuous documentation · Directs team effectively

Critical Fail Triggers:

✗ Fails to call for senior help immediately — manages alone
✗ Does not site two large-bore IV cannulae
✗ Forgets to catheterise bladder before uterotonic therapy
✗ Fails to activate Major Haemorrhage Protocol when EBL >1500mL
✗ Fails to prescribe oxytocin infusion as first-line uterotonic

SAY — Examiner Debrief Prompts:

- EBL reaches 1500mL, BP 72/40. What do you activate and what does that trigger?
- Why does a full bladder worsen uterine atony?
- Senior asks if surgical intervention is needed. What options exist?
- How do you communicate to an extremely distressed partner?

NOTE — Memory Anchor: HELP-ROCC → Help (call immediately) + Establish IV ×2 large-bore + Prescribe Oxytocin infusion (first-line) + Resuscitate + Uterine massage + Catheterise + Crossmatch

STATION 11 — REDUCED FETAL MOVEMENTS

Candidate Brief:

Mrs Clarke, 32, 38 weeks pregnant, reduced movements for 3 days. Tasks: focused obstetric history · initiate assessments · communicate and escalate.

☐ **Immediate Actions:**

☐ Take full obstetric history: gestation, scans, risk factors
☐ Ask specifically: HOW LONG has movement been reduced? (3 days = critical)
☐ Maternal observations: BP, HR, SpO_2, temperature
☐ Auscultate fetal heart with Doppler immediately
☐ Attach CTG monitoring — minimum 20-minute trace
☐ USS if CTG is non-reassuring or clinical concern remains
☐ Escalate to obstetric senior if CTG non-reassuring or reduced movements >24h
☐ Document: gestation, risk factors, fetal heart rate, CTG findings, plan
☐ Do NOT discharge with 3 days reduced movements without CTG + senior review

Layered Actor Script:

🟢 **DEFAULT:** Anxious but calm. Holding her bump. First attendance for this.

🟡 **IF DELAY:** "Should you be checking the heartbeat? My friend said they did that for her."

🔴 **IF NO ESCALATION:** "I looked it up online and it said reduced movements can mean distress. Is mine?"

SAY — ACTOR PROMPT: "She was moving loads last week. Now it's just... quiet. I waited 3 days hoping it would improve."

Hidden Info — reveal only if asked directly:

Duration: 3 days — not just today (critical — prolonged reduction is higher risk)
Normal pattern: Baby was very active — 10+ movements per day
Current count: Maybe 3–4 gentle movements today if she concentrates
Previous scan: Normal growth, normal liquor at 28 weeks
Risk factors: BMI 34, gestational diabetes diagnosed at 28 weeks — only if asked
Other symptoms: No PV bleeding, no pain, no headache, no visual disturbance

Domain (marks)	Criteria
Communication (4)	Introduces + validates concern · Explains FM significance without panic · Explains each investigation · Confirms understanding
History & Risk Assessment (6)	Duration 3 days established · Previous FM pattern · Risk factors: BMI 34, GDM · Associated symptoms · Gestation 38 weeks · Previous growth scan normal
Investigation & Management (6)	Doppler immediately · CTG ≥20 minutes · USS if CTG non-reassuring · Senior escalation (3 days + GDM) · No discharge without CTG + review · Documents CTG interpretation
Safety (4)	3 days = high-risk — not minimised · No reassurance before assessment · Senior escalated · Full documentation

Critical Fail Triggers:

✗ Reassures mother without performing CTG or Doppler first
✗ Fails to establish that reduced movements have lasted 3 days
✗ Misses gestational diabetes as risk factor when asked
✗ Discharges without CTG and senior review

SAY — Examiner Debrief Prompts:

- CTG: baseline 150bpm, reduced variability, no accelerations. How do you classify this?
- She asks: is my baby going to be alright? What do you say?
- Why does 3 days duration matter vs reduced movements today only?
- Senior asks you to prepare for emergency caesarean. What do you do immediately?

NOTE — Memory Anchor: DAME-USS → Duration (3 days critical) + Auscultate Doppler + Monitor CTG (minimum 20 min) + Escalate (senior + USS if non-reassuring)

THINK — STATION 12 — SELF-HARM RISK ASSESSMENT

Candidate Brief:

Sam, 22, brought to ED with superficial forearm cuts. Cooperative. Tasks: therapeutic rapport · structured self-harm risk assessment · safety plan and escalation. Approach with warmth. Do NOT be judgemental.

☐ **Immediate Actions:**

- ☐ Ensure physical safety: wounds dressed, vitals stable
- ☐ Establish privacy — ask friend to wait outside initially
- ☐ Build rapport before any formal assessment — name, how they feel now
- ☐ Explore trigger using RRSS: Recent event, Reason (intent), Seriousness, Safeguards
- ☐ Ask directly but sensitively about suicidal ideation, plan, means, intent
- ☐ Explore protective factors: relationships, work, reasons for living
- ☐ Complete structured risk assessment and document risk level + protective factors
- ☐ Do not discharge without psychiatric review or crisis team plan
- ☐ Formulate safety plan: who to call, what to do if urge returns

Layered Actor Script:

🟢 **DEFAULT:** Quiet. Looks at floor. Short answers initially. Not hostile.

🟡 **IF DELAY:** "It just felt like the only way to feel something."

🔴 **IF NO ESCALATION:** "You're just going to tell me I'm attention-seeking, aren't you." Shuts down.

SAY — ACTOR PROMPT: "I'm fine. It's not a big deal. Can I just go home?"

Hidden Info — reveal only if asked directly:

Method: Cut forearms with razor — deliberate, not accidental (ask gently)
Intent: No intent to die — wanted to relieve emotional pain
Trigger: Partner of 3 years left me yesterday
Previous episodes: Twice before, aged 17 — never told anyone
Current mental state: Low mood 3 weeks, poor sleep, not eating well
Protective factors: Close friend who brought me in. Still goes to work.
Suicidal ideation: Sometimes thinks about not waking up — but no plan, no means

Domain (marks)	Criteria
Communication (6)	Introduces warmly (not formal first) · Creates private calm environment · Open non-judgemental language · No shock/disgust/minimisation · Validates: "That sounds incredibly painful" · Checks-in: "Is it OK to keep talking?"
Risk Assessment (8)	Explores trigger (relationship breakdown) · Establishes intent (pain relief, not death) · Previous self-harm: age 17 never disclosed · Suicidal ideation/plan/means asked sensitively · Low mood + sleep + appetite 3 weeks · Protective factors: friend, work, no plan · Fleeting thoughts, no active plan · RRSS framework used
Management (4)	No discharge without psychiatric/crisis review · Safety plan collaboratively formed · Follow-up: IAPT/crisis/GP · Friend involved with consent

Domain (marks)	Criteria
Safety (2)	Documents risk level, intent, plan, protective factors · Escalates to psychiatric liaison

Critical Fail Triggers:

✗ Immediately asks "did you want to kill yourself" without building rapport

✗ Discharges without psychiatric review or crisis plan

✗ Reacts with shock or uses language implying blame

✗ Fails to ask about suicidal ideation, plan or means at any point

✗ Fails to document risk level, protective factors and follow-up plan

SAY — Examiner Debrief Prompts:

- Sam denies suicidal intent but you feel uncertain. What do you do?
- Why is asking directly about suicide not "planting the idea"?
- Sam asks to see the friend now. What do you consider before agreeing?
- What does a safety plan include and who collaborates on it?

NOTE — Memory Anchor: RRSS-PD → Recent event + Reason (intent) + Seriousness + Safeguards + Protective factors → Safety plan + Psychiatric review + Document (risk + protective factors + follow-up + who informed)

STATION 13 — ALCOHOL WITHDRAWAL (CIWA-Ar)

Candidate Brief:

Mr Hughes, 48, admitted for elective procedure (postponed). Now sweating, tremulous, agitated. Last alcohol 36 hours ago. Tasks: recognise and assess with CIWA-Ar · safe management including pharmacological · communicate and escalate.

☐ **Immediate Actions:**

☐ CIWA-Ar assessment: 10 items including tremor, sweating, anxiety, nausea, perceptual disturbances

☐ Vitals: HR, BP, Temperature, SpO_2 — establish baseline

☐ IV access + bloods: FBC, U&E, LFTs, glucose, magnesium, thiamine

☐ IV Pabrinex (thiamine) BEFORE any glucose — prevent Wernicke's encephalopathy

☐ Chlordiazepoxide reducing regimen prescribed (PRN if CIWA-guided, fixed if severe)

☐ Oral/IV fluids if vomiting or haemodynamically compromised

☐ Hourly observations + repeat CIWA scoring

☐ Escalate to senior if CIWA >15, seizure, or haemodynamic instability

☐ Alert anaesthetic/ICU given previous withdrawal seizure history

Layered Actor Script:

🟢 **DEFAULT:** Sweating heavily. Hands trembling visibly. Irritable but cooperative.

🟡 **IF DELAY:** "Doctor, I feel like my skin is crawling. I can't sit still. Is this normal after stopping?"

🔴 **IF NO ESCALATION:** "I think I'm going to be sick... everything feels like it's shaking."

SAY — ACTOR PROMPT: "I only have a few drinks a day. I don't understand why I feel so terrible."

Hidden Info — reveal only if asked directly:
Actual alcohol intake: 15–20 units per day for 5 years — only if asked specifically
Previous withdrawal: Had a seizure once when tried to stop before
Last drink: 36 hours ago — confirms withdrawal timeline
CIWA score: Score 14 (moderate) — if candidate asks for specific features
Other medical history: Known hypertension, on amlodipine
Allergies: NKDA

Domain (marks)	Criteria
Communication (4)	No judgement about alcohol use · Explains AWS in plain language · Non-judgemental and empathetic · Explains each medication
Assessment (6)	CIWA-Ar 10 domains described/calculated · True intake: 15–20 units/day (hidden) · Previous seizure = high-risk · Vitals documented · CIWA ≈14 (moderate) · Wernicke's risk recognised
Management (6)	IV Pabrinex BEFORE glucose · Chlordiazepoxide reducing regimen · IV fluids · Hourly obs + repeat CIWA · Senior escalated (previous seizure) · ICU/anaesthetic alerted
Safety (4)	No glucose-containing fluids before thiamine · No diazepam alone without monitoring · Escalated early · CIWA + medications documented

Critical Fail Triggers:

✗ Gives IV glucose BEFORE IV Pabrinex (thiamine) — precipitates Wernicke's encephalopathy

✗ Fails to identify previous withdrawal seizure history when asked

✗ Does not escalate despite CIWA >10 and previous seizure history

✗ Fails to prescribe thiamine at all

SAY — Examiner Debrief Prompts:

- Why must thiamine be given before glucose? What does it prevent?
- CIWA score is 14. Is that mild, moderate or severe? What does it change?
- He has a seizure on the ward. What do you do in the next 60 seconds?
- He asks if he needs to stop drinking permanently. How do you approach this?

NOTE — Memory Anchor: THICCS-P → Thiamine IV (Pabrinex) BEFORE glucose + CIWA score + High-risk features (prev seizure) + Chlordiazepoxide + Close monitoring + Senior if seizure risk + Pabrinex (examiners expect this term)

STATION 14 — CONSENT FOR LUMBAR PUNCTURE

Candidate Brief:

Mr Shah, 34, admitted with severe headache, photophobia, neck stiffness. CT head normal. Tasks: explain indication · describe procedure + risks + alternatives · obtain valid informed consent.

☐ **Immediate Actions:**

☐ Introduce self + confirm patient identity and capacity

☐ Explain indication: exclude bacterial meningitis / SAH

☐ Explain procedure: positioning, local anaesthetic, needle at L3/4 or L4/5

☐ Explain risks: post-LP headache (MOST COMMON), infection, bleeding, nerve damage (rare), failure

☐ Explain benefits: essential diagnostic information, guides antibiotic treatment

☐ Explain alternatives and consequences of refusal

☐ Check latex allergy — use latex-free equipment

☐ Answer questions — address paralysis misconception

☐ Document consent: procedure, risks explained, questions answered, patient consented voluntarily

Layered Actor Script:

🟢 **DEFAULT:** Anxious. Headache severe. Cooperative but worried about needle in back.

🟡 **IF DELAY:** "A headache from a headache procedure? How does that make sense?" (Sceptical)

🔴 **IF NO ESCALATION:** "Wait — you said you have to tell me all the risks. What are you not telling me?"

SAY — ACTOR PROMPT: "What if I just refuse? Can you make me have it? I'm a solicitor — I know my rights."

Hidden Info — reveal only if asked directly:

Why he is worried: Had a friend with chronic back pain after an epidural — only if asked

His understanding: Thinks it might paralyse him — heard things can go wrong with spinal needles

Allergies: ALLERGIC TO LATEX — important for equipment selection

Capacity: Has full capacity — confirms after brief assessment

Religion/belief: No religious objections — not relevant here

Domain (marks)	**Criteria**
Communication (4)	Introduces + confirms capacity · Appropriate to educated patient (solicitor) · Does not rush · Calm when challenged
Consent Content (8)	Indication: exclude meningitis/SAH · Procedure accurately described · Risks: post-LP headache (most common), infection, bleeding, nerve damage, failure · Benefits: definitive diagnosis · Consequences of refusal · Can withdraw consent · Latex allergy addressed · Documents consent
Autonomy & Ethics (4)	Capacity confirmed before proceeding · Consent is voluntary · Right to refuse confirmed + consequences explained · Care not withdrawn if refuses
Safety (4)	No risks skipped or minimised · Paralysis misconception addressed factually · No jargon without checking · Full documentation

Critical Fail Triggers:

✗ Fails to explain post-LP headache as the MOST COMMON risk

✗ Does not address patient's direct question about refusing

✗ Proceeds to document consent without confirming capacity

✗ Misses latex allergy — does not ask or address

SAY — Examiner Debrief Prompts:

- He refuses. What exactly do you do next — step by step?
- He asks: what are the chances of paralysis? How do you answer accurately?
- Why did you check capacity before taking consent?
- He signs but says he's still not sure. Is that valid consent?

NOTE — Memory Anchor: I-BRAVE-A → Indication + Benefits + Risks (post-LP headache MOST COMMON; infection; bleeding; nerve damage; failure) + Alternatives + Voluntary + Extras (latex allergy, capacity) + Document

STATION 15 — INSULIN PRESCRIPTION (VRIII)

Candidate Brief:

Mrs Okafor, 58, T2DM (HbA1c 92), elective laparoscopic cholecystectomy tomorrow, NBM from midnight. Tasks: focused diabetes + medication history · prescribe VRIII safely · explain plan and arrange monitoring.

☐ **Immediate Actions:**

☐ Take full diabetes history: type, duration, medications, HbA1c, recent hypos

☐ Check renal function (creatinine 88 — normal, eGFR >60)

☐ Withhold metformin from midnight — lactic acidosis risk perioperatively

☐ Withhold gliclazide from midnight — hypoglycaemia risk when NBM

☐ Prescribe VRIII: Actrapid/Novorapid + 5% glucose + 0.9% saline with KCl

☐ Select ENHANCED rate scale (HbA1c 92 = poor control)

☐ Hourly blood glucose monitoring while on VRIII

☐ Target glucose range: 6–10 mmol/L perioperatively

☐ Prescribe hypoglycaemia rescue protocol on drug chart

☐ Explain plan: NBM, VRIII, hourly glucose checks, resume normal meds post-op

Layered Actor Script:

🟢 **DEFAULT:** Anxious about surgery. Cooperative. Brings her medication list.

🟡 **IF DELAY:** "I take metformin at home. Is that OK to take with the drip?"

🔴 **IF NO ESCALATION:** "No one has told me what the plan is for my sugars overnight. Should I be worried?"

SAY — ACTOR PROMPT: "My last operation was years ago and my sugars went really high afterwards. I don't want that to happen again."

Hidden Info — reveal only if asked directly:

Current medications: Metformin 1g BD + gliclazide 80mg OD + amlodipine 5mg OD

Metformin guidance: Withhold on day of surgery and 48h post-op (lactic acidosis risk with anaesthesia/contrast)

Allergies: NKDA

Renal function: Creatinine 88 µmol/L — normal, eGFR >60

Previous hypoglycaemia: One episode 6 months ago — treated with oral glucose at home

Weight: 82 kg — relevant for insulin dosing

Domain (marks)	Criteria
Communication (4)	Introduces + explains purpose · Structured medication history · Explains NBM + VRIII plan in plain language · Addresses concern about previous high sugars
Medication Management (6)	Identifies metformin · Withholds with correct rationale (lactic acidosis) · Withholds gliclazide (hypo risk NBM) · Checks renal function · HbA1c 92 = enhanced scale · Hypo rescue prescribed
VRIII Prescribing (6)	Actrapid/Novorapid infusion · 5% glucose infusion (CRITICAL) · 0.9% saline + KCl · Enhanced rate scale · Hourly BG monitoring · Target 6–10 documented
Safety (4)	No VRIII without glucose infusion · No metformin perioperatively · Full documentation · Escalates to diabetes specialist nurse if uncertain

Critical Fail Triggers:

✗ Continues metformin perioperatively without addressing lactic acidosis risk

✗ Prescribes insulin infusion WITHOUT accompanying glucose — hypoglycaemia risk

✗ Fails to arrange hourly blood glucose monitoring

✗ Does not withhold gliclazide when patient is NBM

SAY — Examiner Debrief Prompts:

- BG at midnight is 3.2 mmol/L. What do you do with the VRIII?
- Why must metformin be stopped perioperatively? What is the risk?
- HbA1c is 92. Which rate scale do you use and why?
- She asks when she can restart her normal diabetes medications post-op.

NOTE — Memory Anchor: VRIII-SWIM → Withhold metformin+gliclazide (lactic acidosis) + Rate scale (enhanced if HbA1c >69) + Insulin + Glucose infusion (5% — MUST prescribe together) + Monitor hourly BG

STATION 16 — ECG / DATA INTERPRETATION (Hyperkalaemia)

Candidate Brief:

Mrs Osei, 68, renal outpatient, haemodialysis patient, missed session 3 days ago. Weak and unwell. ECG: peaked T waves V3–V5, widened QRS 130ms. K^+ 7.1, pH 7.28, HCO_3 16. Tasks: interpret ECG + bloods · explain · initiate emergency treatment.

☐ **Immediate Actions:**

☐ Recognise hyperkalaemia: peaked T waves + widened QRS = cardiac emergency

☐ IV calcium gluconate 10% 10mL over 2–3 minutes IMMEDIATELY (membrane stabilisation)

☐ Continuous cardiac monitoring throughout

☐ Insulin 10 units Actrapid + 50mL 50% glucose IV (intracellular K+ shift)

☐ Salbutamol 10–20mg nebulised (additional K+ shift)

☐ Calcium resonium PO or sodium zirconium cyclosilicate (K+ removal)

☐ Escalate urgently to renal team for emergency dialysis

Layered Actor Script:

🟢 **DEFAULT:** Weak, slightly confused. Cooperative but frightened.

🟡 **IF DELAY:** "My heart feels like it's fluttering... is that from my kidneys?"

🔴 **IF NO ESCALATION:** "I feel really strange. Doctor, is my heart okay?" Grips chest lightly.

SAY — ACTOR PROMPT: "Something doesn't feel right. I feel very heavy and weak."

Hidden Info — reveal only if asked directly:

Missed dialysis: Missed session 3 days ago — only if asked directly

Diet: Ate bananas and tomatoes yesterday (high-potassium foods)

Medications: Sodium bicarbonate and cinacalcet — may have missed doses

Previous K+ baseline: Usually 5.2–5.6 between dialysis sessions

Domain (marks)	Criteria
Communication (4)	Introduces + confirms ID · Explains ECG + bloods in plain language ("dangerously high potassium") · Explains each step · Conveys urgency without panic
ECG & Data Interpretation (6)	Peaked T waves V3–V5 identified · Widened QRS 130ms · Hyperkalaemia diagnosed (ECG + K+ 7.1) · Metabolic acidosis (pH 7.28, HCO3 16) · Missed dialysis correlated · Critical threshold K+ ≥6.5 with ECG = emergency
Management (6)	Ca gluconate FIRST (membrane stabilisation before K+ lowering) · Insulin + 50% glucose · Salbutamol nebuliser · K+ removal: resonium/sodium zirconium · Urgent renal for emergency dialysis · Continuous cardiac monitoring
Safety (4)	No delay in calcium gluconate · No insulin without glucose · Urgent renal escalation · Documents K+/ECG/treatment/times

Critical Fail Triggers:

✗ Fails to identify peaked T waves or widened QRS on ECG

✗ Does NOT give calcium gluconate 10% 10mL IV as FIRST step — gives insulin first (ventricular arrhythmia risk)

✗ Prescribes insulin WITHOUT accompanying glucose infusion

✗ Fails to escalate to renal team for emergency dialysis

SAY — Examiner Debrief Prompts:

- Why give calcium gluconate before insulin — what does each drug do?
- K+ is 7.1 and patient looks reasonably well. Does appearance change your urgency?
- What dietary advice do you give before discharge?
- Which calcium salt do you use and why — gluconate vs chloride?

NOTE — Memory Anchor: HYPERK-R → Halt arrhythmia (Ca gluconate 10% 10mL IV over 2–3 min — preferred over chloride) + Yield K+ into cells (insulin+glucose) + Push K+ out (resonium) + Escalate Renal + Keep monitoring + Remove K+ (resonium/dialysis if refractory)

STATION 17 — TELEPHONE CONSULTATION (Possible ACS)

Candidate Brief:

You are on-call FY2 at 22:30. Mr Patel, 61, calls from home with central chest tightness 20 minutes. Tasks: safe telephone consultation · assess red flags remotely · safe clinical decision and documentation. No face-to-face possible. Do NOT advise driving.

☐ **Immediate Actions:**

☐ Identify yourself: name, role, grade

☐ Confirm patient identity: full name, DOB, home address

☐ Establish reason for call: onset, site, quality, radiation, duration

☐ Ask red flags: sweating, nausea, arm/jaw pain, breathlessness, previous cardiac history

☐ DO NOT advise driving or taking a taxi to hospital

☐ Advise patient to call 999 immediately — ACS until proven otherwise

☐ Advise: chew aspirin 300mg if not already taken and no allergy

☐ Advise: sit or lie down, do not exert, wife stays with him

☐ Stay on line or agree callback in 5 minutes to confirm 999 called

☐ Document: time of call, content, advice given, action taken, safety-net

Layered Actor Script:

🟢 **DEFAULT:** Slightly breathless on phone. Short sentences. Playing down symptoms.

🟡 **IF DELAY:** "I feel a bit sick now and my left arm has gone numb and tingly."

🔴 **IF NO ESCALATION:** "Are you sure? I'm feeling dizzy now... My wife is here with me." Sounds frightened.

SAY — ACTOR PROMPT: "My wife said I should call. I didn't want to bother anyone, especially so late."

Hidden Info — reveal only if asked directly:

Pain radiation: Radiating to left arm and jaw — only if directly asked

Sweating: Yes — sweating heavily despite sitting still

Previous cardiac history: Had a heart attack 2 years ago — stents inserted

Medications: Aspirin 75mg, bisoprolol, ramipril — no GTN spray

Someone with him: Wife is at home, can call 999

Allergies: NKDA

Domain (marks)	Criteria
Communication (6)	Identifies self + role at start · Confirms patient ID (name/DOB/address) · Speaks clearly/calmly · Focused questions · Summarises back before advising · Documents call
Clinical Assessment (6)	Onset/site/quality/duration · Radiation: left arm + jaw (high-risk pattern) · Associated features: sweating/nausea · High-risk history: NSTEMI + stents · Currently on aspirin — checks additional 300mg safety · ACS pattern identified
Management (4)	Advises 999 (not driving) · Advises chewing aspirin 300mg (ACS protocol) · Stay still/sit/lie/no exertion · Callback in 5 min or stays on line
Safety (4)	ACS urgency recognised · No false reassurance · SBAR documentation · Escalates if uncertain

Critical Fail Triggers:

✗ Advises patient to DRIVE or take a taxi to hospital — cardiac event at wheel

✗ Tells patient to wait until GP surgery opens

✗ Gives false reassurance without completing full symptom assessment

✗ Fails to confirm patient identity at the start of the call

✗ Fails to document the call

SAY — Examiner Debrief Prompts:

- Why is telling him to drive potentially more dangerous than 999?
- He says the pain has settled now. Does that change your advice?
- What exactly do you document and why does it have medico-legal significance?
- Could this have been managed without calling 999? What threshold applies?

NOTE — Memory Anchor: IRACE-D → Identify (self + patient) + Red flags + Assess history + Call 999 + Explain (do NOT advise driving) + Document (time, advice, outcome)

SAY — STATION 18 — ANGRY RELATIVE (Duty of Candour)

Candidate Brief:

Mrs Clarke, 55, daughter of Mr Clarke, 82 (hip fracture). She is unhappy about a 6-hour ED wait and a sacral pressure sore. Tasks: manage professionally and compassionately · Duty of Candour · clear plan + complaints pathway.

☐ **Immediate Actions:**

☐ Find a private room IMMEDIATELY before beginning any conversation
☐ Introduce self and role clearly
☐ Allow relative to speak fully without interruption
☐ Acknowledge her concerns explicitly BEFORE explaining anything
☐ Deliver CLEAR, UNCONDITIONAL apology: "I am sorry that this happened"
☐ Do NOT use conditional language: avoid "I'm sorry you feel..."
☐ Do NOT be defensive or blame colleagues or other departments
☐ Do NOT speculate about disciplinary outcomes
☐ Explain factually what is known — do not speculate
☐ Outline what is being done: wound care, pressure relief, hip surgery plan
☐ Offer PALS and formal complaints pathway
☐ Offer written follow-up within agreed timeframe
☐ Document: time, concerns raised, what was said, plan agreed

Layered Actor Script:

🟢 **DEFAULT:** Angry, upset, determined. Clearly has been building up to this conversation.

🟡 **IF DELAY:** "I've been trying to speak to someone for hours. No one has bothered to explain anything."

🔴 **IF NO ESCALATION:** "If you can't give me answers I'm going to make a formal complaint TODAY."

SAY — ACTOR PROMPT: "I just want someone to say sorry and tell me it won't happen to someone else."

Hidden Info — reveal only if asked directly:

Father's condition: Stable. Hip surgery scheduled for tomorrow morning.
Pressure sore: Grade 2 sacral — wound care team informed
Formal complaint: No formal complaint yet — wanted to speak first
Father's wishes: Mr Clarke has capacity and asked his daughter to come on his behalf
What she wants: Someone to say sorry and know it won't happen to others

Domain (marks)	**Criteria**
Communication (8)	Private space found first · Allows full speech without interruption · Uses "Mrs Clarke" throughout · No defensive language · Acknowledges distress explicitly · Clear unconditional apology · Factual explanation without speculation · Checks understanding
Duty of Candour (6)	Acknowledges something went wrong (6h wait, pressure sore) · Unconditional apology (not "sorry you feel") · Explains pressure sore management · Outlines investigation process · Provides PALS + complaints pathway · Written follow-up offered
Safety (6)	No promises about investigation outcome · No speculation about disciplinary · Professional composure maintained · Sets calm boundary if threatening · No other patient information disclosed · Full documentation

Critical Fail Triggers:

X "I'm sorry you feel that way" — CONDITIONAL apology (instant fail)
X Being defensive, dismissive or blaming other team members
X Making promises about the outcome of any investigation
X Discussing another patient's confidential information
X Conducting conversation in a public area without privacy

SAY — Examiner Debrief Prompts:

- What is the difference between a genuine apology and a conditional one? Why does it matter legally?
- She asks: are you saying the nurse was negligent? How do you respond?
- She starts crying mid-conversation. What do you do?
- What would you document after this, and who else would you inform and when?

NOTE — Memory Anchor: LAAPED → Listen + Apologise unconditionally ("I am sorry this happened" — NOT "I'm sorry you feel...") + Acknowledge + Explain (factual) + Investigate (inform of process) + Plan + Document

Part 2 Rapid Reference — Stations 10–18

Stn	Station	Memory Anchor	Key Hidden Info	Critical Fail
10	PPH	HELP-ROCC: Help+IV×2+Oxytocin+Resus+Uterine massage+Catheterise+Crossmatch	EBL 1100mL ongoing · bladder not catheterised	No senior call · no oxytocin infusion · no catheter
11	Reduced FM	DAME-USS: Duration(3d)+Auscultate+Monitor CTG(20min)+Escalate+USS	Duration 3 days · GDM · BMI 34	Reassure without CTG · miss 3-day duration
12	Self-Harm	RRSS-PD: Recent+Reason+Seriousness+Safeguards+Protective→Safety plan+Document	Prev self-harm age 17 · fleeting SI no plan	Rapport not built first · discharge without psych review
13	Alcohol WD	THICCS-P: Pabrinex BEFORE glucose+CIWA+Chlordiazepoxide+Monitor+Senior	15–20 units/day · prev seizure · CIWA 14	Glucose before thiamine · miss seizure history
14	Consent LP	I-BRAVE-A: Indication+Benefits+Risks+Alternatives+Voluntary+Extras+Document	Latex allergy · paralysis misconception	Miss post-LP headache (most common) · miss latex allergy

Stn	Station	Memory Anchor	Key Hidden Info	Critical Fail
15	Insulin VRIII	VRIII-SWIM: Withhold metformin/glicl+Rate scale+Insulin+Glucose+ Monitor hourly	Metformin on med list · HbA1c 92 = enhanced scale	Insulin without glucose · continue metformin periop
16	ECG/Hyp erk	HYPERK-R: Ca gluconate FIRST+Insulin+glucose +Resonium+Renal escalation	Missed dialysis 3 days · high-K+ diet	Insulin before calcium gluconate · no renal escalation
17	Telephone	IRACE-D: Identify+Red flags+Assess+Call 999+Explain(NO driving)+Document	Jaw radiation · prev MI + stents · no GTN	Advise driving · false reassurance · no documentation
18	Angry Relative	LAAPED: Listen+Apologise unconditionally+Acknow ledge+Explain+Investig ate+Plan+Document	Grade 2 pressure sore · father has capacity	Conditional apology · defensive/blame · no private space

Critical Safety Summary — 5 Deadly Sequences

5 Deadly Prescribing/Treatment Sequences:
Stn 5: CAP antibiotics for 7 days (must be 5) — incorrect duration
Stn 13: IV glucose BEFORE thiamine → Wernicke's encephalopathy
Stn 15: Insulin without glucose infusion (VRIII) → profound hypoglycaemia
Stn 16: Insulin before calcium gluconate → ventricular arrhythmia
Stn 17: Advise patient to drive to hospital → cardiac event at wheel

Station	Correct Sequence	Wrong Sequence
Stn 8 Sepsis	Blood cultures → THEN antibiotics	Antibiotics first (destroys culture evidence)
Stn 13 Alcohol WD	Thiamine (Pabrinex) → THEN glucose	Glucose first → Wernicke's
Stn 15 VRIII	Insulin + glucose infusion TOGETHER	Insulin alone → hypoglycaemia
Stn 16 Hyperkalaemia	Calcium gluconate → THEN insulin + glucose	Insulin first → arrhythmia risk
Stn 7 Anaphylaxis	Adrenaline IM → THEN chlorphenamine + hydrocortisone	Antihistamine first → fails to address anaphylaxis
Stn 6 Stroke	CT head → THEN aspirin	Aspirin before CT → haemorrhage risk

NOTE — All 18 Memory Anchors — Complete Reference

Stn	Station	Anchor	Full Mnemonic
1	Chest Pain	AMEN	ABC + Monitor + ECG within 10min + eNquire → Aspirin + Escalate + NEWS2
2	Paeds Fever	SAFE-D	SpO_2 + Assess WOB + Fever + Escalate + Dehydration + DON'T FORGET RASH
3	Bad News	SPIKES+N URSE	Setting → Perception → Invitation → Knowledge → Empathy (NURSE) → Strategy
4	Capacity	URWC	Understand + Retain + Weigh + Communicate → Document + Escalate if absent
5	Drug Chart	DDRF-AR+5DAYS	Drug + Dose(renal) + Route + Freq + Allergy(reaction type) + Review + Duration(5 days)
6	Stroke	FAST-CT+INR	FAST + Glucose + CT head → Stroke team → Thrombolysis window → Check INR
7	Anaphylaxi s	AIR	Adrenaline IM 0.5mg 1:1000 → In anterolateral thigh → Repeat 5 min + O_2 + Fluids
8	Sepsis	Sepsis-6+TIME ZERO	Cultures+Lactate+Urine (TAKE) → Antibiotics+Fluids+O_2 (GIVE) → Escalate + Document time zero
9	Bronchioliti s	SAFE-B	SpO_2 + Assess + Feed + Escalate + Supportive (NO suction/bronchodilators/steroids)
10	PPH	HELP-ROCC	Help + IV×2 + Oxytocin infusion + Resuscitate + Uterine massage + Catheterise + Crossmatch
11	Reduced FM	DAME-USS	Duration(3d) + Auscultate Doppler + Monitor CTG(20min) + Escalate + USS if non-reassuring
12	Self-Harm	RRSS-PD	Recent + Reason + Seriousness + Safeguards + Protective → Safety plan + Document
13	Alcohol WD	THICCS-P	Thiamine (Pabrinex) BEFORE glucose + CIWA + High-risk + Chlordiazepoxide + Close monitoring + Senior
14	Consent LP	I-BRAVE-A	Indication + Benefits + Risks (post-LP headache MOST COMMON) + Alternatives + Voluntary + Extras + Document
15	Insulin VRIII	VRIII-SWIM	Withhold metformin+gliclazide + Rate scale(enhanced if HbA1c >69) + Insulin + Glucose(MUST) + Monitor hourly
16	ECG/Hype rk	HYPERK-R	Ca gluconate FIRST + Yield K+ (insulin+glucose) + Push out (resonium) + Escalate Renal + Keep monitoring
17	Telephone	IRACE-D	Identify + Red flags + Assess + Call 999 + Explain(NO driving) + Document
18	Angry Relative	LAAPED	Listen + Apologise unconditionally + Acknowledge + Explain + Investigate + Plan + Document

✓ Universal Documentation Checklist — Every Station

Complete before leaving every station:

☐ Patient name, DOB, hospital number · ☐ Date and TIME · ☐ Key history findings

☐ Examination findings · ☐ Investigations ordered + why · ☐ Management: drugs/doses/routes/durations

☐ Escalation: who was informed and when · ☐ Safety-netting advice given

☐ Your name, signature, GMC number, bleep, designation

Universal Rules — Every Station:

ABC before anything else (all emergencies) · Introduce + confirm ID (all stations) · Safety-net before any discharge · Escalate early

Allergy check BEFORE prescribing · No routine O_2 without SpO_2 check · No aspirin before CT (stroke) · Calcium gluconate BEFORE insulin (hyperkalaemia)

Thiamine BEFORE glucose (alcohol WD) · Blood cultures BEFORE antibiotics (sepsis) · Unconditional apology only (candour) · Never advise driving — always 999

APPENDIX 3D · MOCK OSCE PERFORMANCE GUIDE

How to Use Stations · Weak vs Strong Candidate · When It Goes Wrong · 7-Day Sprint Plan · Model Performances

AMaC (A. Mansour and Colleagues) · PLAB 2 Master Series · Volume 3

Abbreviations used in this appendix: BNF British National Formulary · CAP Community-Acquired Pneumonia · CIWA Clinical Institute Withdrawal Assessment · CTG Cardiotocography · CURB-65 CURB-65 pneumonia severity score · DKA Diabetic Ketoacidosis · EBL Estimated Blood Loss · IUGR Intrauterine Growth Restriction · LP Lumbar Puncture · MSE Mental State Examination · NEWS2 National Early Warning Score 2 · PCI Percutaneous Coronary Intervention · PE Pulmonary Embolism · PPH Postpartum Haemorrhage · RCUK Resuscitation Council UK · SAH Subarachnoid Haemorrhage · UKMLA UK Medical Licensing Assessment · VRIII Variable Rate Intravenous Insulin Infusion

How to Use These 18 Mock Stations

These are rehearsal tools, not reading exercises. A station read passively is worth very little. A station performed, timed, recorded, and self-audited is worth more than a week of passive revision.

Mode	Setup	How to Do It
Solo Practice	Timer · Phone camera	Read brief. Start timer. Speak aloud — every thought, action, reasoning step. Record yourself. Play back and mark against the marking scheme. Most candidates are shocked by how much they silently think rather than verbalise.
Paired Practice	2 people · Timer · Full materials	Candidate reads brief only. Actor reads the layered script AND all hidden information. Actor does NOT reveal hidden info unless asked directly — this is crucial. After 8 minutes, actor gives feedback using the marking scheme. Swap roles.
Group Circuit	4–6 people · Full circuit	Assign roles: candidates rotate, actors stay. Use 8-minute timings with 2-minute reading time between stations. Debrief after every 3 stations using the rapid reference tables.
Exam Simulation	Final week only	No prep after brief is handed over. No notes. No chapter re-reading. This simulates real exam stress. The errors you make here are the ones to fix before exam day.

Actor Rules — Critical:

1. Do NOT reveal hidden information unless candidate asks directly and specifically.

2. Follow the layered script: start cooperative (green), escalate if candidate delays or mismanages.

3. Stay in character. If candidate makes an error, let it happen — the debrief addresses it.

4. Feedback order: what they did well → what lost marks → what would have failed the station.

Weak vs Strong Candidate — 5 Critical Moments

These are the moments where most candidates lose marks. Not on clinical knowledge. On performance. The difference is often a single sentence.

1. Opening the Station

Scenario: Candidate enters. Patient diaphoretic, clutching chest. Chest pain station.

✗ Weak Candidate	✓ Strong Candidate
Walks in, sits down.	**Knocks, enters, eye contact, washes hands visibly. Scans patient.**
Asks: "So what seems to be the problem?"	**Hello, I'm Dr Ali, one of the doctors. Can I confirm your name and date of birth? I can see you're in discomfort — I'm going to check your vital signs while we talk — is that okay?**
Starts taking history.	**Attaches monitoring while asking first question.**

✓ **Lesson:** The first 30 seconds determine the examiner's impression. Introduce, confirm ID, acknowledge distress, state immediate priority. This scores 2–3 marks before a single clinical word.

Mark Impact: Communication domain: 0/4 (weak) vs 4/4 (strong)

2. Patient Refuses Treatment

Scenario: 78-year-old refuses insulin. Blood glucose 24 mmol/L.

✗ Weak Candidate	✓ Strong Candidate
Mr Jones, you really need this insulin. Without it you could go into a coma.	**I can hear you're worried, and I want to understand exactly why. Can you tell me what concerns you most about the insulin?**
I strongly advise you to accept the treatment.	**(After hearing hypo fear): That makes complete sense. A hypoglycaemic episode is frightening. I want to address that concern directly.**
If you refuse I'll have to get my consultant.	**(After capacity assessment): You have the right to make this decision. I need to make sure you fully understand the risks so your choice is informed.**

✓ **Lesson:** The examiner watches HOW you handle refusal. Non-coercion, empathy, and a proper capacity assessment score full marks. Persuasion without these scores very little.

Mark Impact: Capacity domain: 1/8 (weak) vs 8/8 (strong)

3. Breaking Bad News — The Delivery Moment

Scenario: Explaining breast cancer diagnosis. Patient expects good news.

✗ Weak Candidate	✓ Strong Candidate

The biopsy shows the lump is malignant. It's a cancer called invasive ductal carcinoma.	**Before I share the results, I want to check — what has been going through your mind since the biopsy?**
(Immediately continues): The good news is we have many treatment options available today...	**(Warning shot): The news I have to share is not the news we were hoping for.**
	(PAUSE. Full silence. Wait for patient response before continuing.)

✓ **Lesson:** The pause after delivering the diagnosis is not empty time. It is the most important clinical act in a breaking bad news station. Continuing to speak while a patient processes a cancer diagnosis is one of the most common fail triggers.
Mark Impact: Communication domain: 2/10 (weak) vs 9/10 (strong)

4. Unwell Patient Mid-Consultation

Scenario: History taking. Patient mid-sentence becomes diaphoretic and short of breath.

✗ Weak Candidate	✓ Strong Candidate
Continues history: "So you mentioned the pain started three hours ago..."	**Immediately: "I'm going to stop our conversation — you don't look well. I'm checking your vital signs now."**
Asks more history questions.	**ABCDE out loud: "Airway patent. Breathing — elevated rate, increased work of breathing. Circulation — pulse rapid and thready. I need to call for help immediately."**
Eventually: "I think we need to get some tests done."	**Can someone bring the emergency trolley? I need senior support at bedside now.**

✓ **Lesson:** Continuing to take a history while a patient deteriorates is an automatic safety fail. This is the most frequent reason clinically knowledgeable candidates fail PLAB 2.
Mark Impact: Safety domain: 0/4 (weak) — station fail. Strong: 4/4.

5. Data Interpretation — Silence vs Verbalisation

Scenario: ECG handed over. Peaked T waves, wide QRS. Dialysis patient missed 3 sessions.

✗ Weak Candidate	✓ Strong Candidate
(Stares at ECG silently for 30 seconds).	**Rate — 72. Rhythm — regular. P waves present. PR interval normal. QRS widened — approximately 140 milliseconds. T waves — strikingly peaked in V3–V5.**
I think there might be some changes here.	**The combination of peaked T waves and widened QRS in a dialysis patient = hyperkalaemia until proven otherwise. This is a cardiac emergency.**

I would like to get some bloods.	**First action: IV calcium gluconate 10% 10mL over 2–3 minutes. Calling for immediate senior and cardiac monitoring now.**

✓ **Lesson:** "If you don't say it, it doesn't exist." Silence scores zero. The examiner cannot mark reasoning they cannot hear. Talk through every step, including normal findings.
Mark Impact: Clinical domain: 0/8 (weak) vs 8/8 (strong)

When It Goes Wrong — Pass Strategy Scripts

Every candidate will have at least one bad station. What separates passing candidates is not that they never panic — it is that they have a recovery system.

You blank — mind goes empty	✗ **Do NOT:** "Stare in silence. Say I'm sorry, I can't remember." ✓ **Do this:** **"I want to make sure I focus on what matters most to you. Can I just check — what was your main concern today?" (ICE always resets any station and buys thinking time.)** **Why:** *ICE is always safe. Examiners see patient-centredness, not panic.* **Mark impact:** Recovers ICE marks (2–4). Station not lost.
You made a clinical error mid-station	✗ **Do NOT:** Continue as if nothing happened. Or over-apologise repeatedly. ✓ **Do this:** **"I want to correct something I said a moment ago — I said [X] but the correct answer is [Y]. I want to make sure you have accurate information." Then continue normally.** **Why:** *Self-correction is a professional behaviour. Examiners score this positively.* **Mark impact:** Professionalism domain maintained.
The actor is uncooperative	✗ **Do NOT:** Argue. Repeat yourself louder. Get visibly flustered. ✓ **Do this:** **"I can see this is really upsetting. I don't want to argue — I want to understand. Can you help me understand what worries you most?" (BRIDGE: don't argue, bridge.)** **Why:** *Uncooperative actors are a deliberate examiner tool. The station tests how you handle difficulty.* **Mark impact:** Communication domain maintained or improved.
You run out of time	✗ **Do NOT:** Keep talking past the bell. Rush through everything at double speed. ✓ **Do this:** **At 7:00, regardless of where you are: "To summarise — [one sentence]. My plan is [one sentence]. If anything worries you — [safety-net]. Any questions?"** TIP — **Why:** *A structured 60-second close scores safety-net (1–2), summary (1), and closure (1) marks.* **Mark impact:** Recovers 3–4 marks even from a chaotic station.
Examiner debrief question you can't answer	✗ **Do NOT:** Guess confidently. Say "I don't know" and stop. ✓ **Do this:** **"I'm not certain of the exact dose/protocol. I would check the BNF and confirm with my senior. What I do know is that the clinical priority here is [state principle]."** TIP — **Why:** *Uncertainty with appropriate escalation = safe behaviour. Guessing with false confidence = unsafe.* **Mark impact:** Partial credit in clinical reasoning. Safety domain maintained.

Patient deteriorates mid-station	✗ **Do NOT:** Continue the history. Finish the question you were asking. ✓ **Do this:** **"I need to stop. You don't look well. I'm initiating ABCDE assessment now." Then work through it aloud.** TIP — **Why:** *This is the number one safety test. Any delay = safety domain fail. Speed of recognition matters.* **Mark impact:** Safety domain: 4/4. Station saved even if history incomplete.
After a bad station	✗ **Do NOT:** Analyse what you should have said. Carry the feeling into the next station. ✓ **Do this:** **Three slow breaths. Say to yourself: "That station is finished. My score there is fixed. This brief is a new station. I start fresh." Read next brief carefully.** TIP — **Why:** *Cognitive carry-over from a bad station is the most common cause of multiple station failures.* **Mark impact:** Prevents cascade failure across the circuit.

Final Sprint — 7-Day Study Plan (Volume 3 Focus)

This plan assumes you have worked through Volumes 1 and 2. If not, complete Volume 1 communication chapters first — examination technique without consultation skills will not pass PLAB 2.

Each day: Morning = new content. Afternoon = mock practice. Evening = rapid review only. No new content after 8pm.

Day	Morning (2 hrs)	Afternoon (2 hrs)	Evening (45 min)
Day 1	CH57 (Exam foundation) · CH58 (CVS + Resp exam) · App 3A (Timing maps)	Solo practice: Mock Station 1 (Chest Pain) · Record yourself · Self-audit checklist	App 1A (Tier 1 core) · App 1B (Instant-fail behaviours) · No new content
Day 2	CH59 (Abdominal/Thyroid exam) · CH60 (Neurological) · CH61 (GALS/MSK)	Paired practice: Mock Station 2 (Paeds fever) · Station 3 (Bad news) · Debrief each	Review self-audit findings · Drill weakest mnemonic from each chapter
Day 3	CH62 (MSE) · CH63 (Cannulation/ABG) · CH64 (Catheterisation) · CH65 (Suturing)	Station 4 (Capacity) · Station 5 (Drug chart) · Station 6 (Stroke) · Timed	App 2F (Instant-Fail Behaviours) · App 2E (Prescribing safety) · SADMAN + VRIII
Day 4	CH66 (Airway/O2) · CH67 (Prescribing) · CH68 (High-risk drugs) · CH69 (Thinking aloud)	Station 7 (Anaphylaxis) · Station 8 (Sepsis) · Station 9 (Bronchiolitis)	App 2D (Normal values) · Critical values · ACID-ID checklist
Day 5	CH70 (ECG/ABG) · CH71 (CXR) · CH72 (Blood tests) · App 3H (Mark sheet + UKMLA)	App 3B: Stations 10–13 · Full timed circuit · No prep after reading brief	Weak vs Strong comparisons in this appendix · Identify your own patterns
Day 6	App 3C: Stations 14–18 · Full timed circuit · Review all marking schemes afternoon	Target 3 weakest stations from days 1–5 · Re-run with fresh focus · Note improvement	App 3E/3E/3F (Safeguarding · NHS vocab · UK culture) · 30 min max
Day 7	App 1A (1-Page OSCE Weapon) + App 1D (Micro-Summary) ONLY · No new chapters	Light review: 5 stations you feel least confident about · Read, do not drill	Prepare bag (Vol 1 App 1E checklist) · Sleep by 10pm · You are ready

Day 7 Rule: No new content on the day before your exam. Your brain needs consolidation time, not new information. Read only what you already know. Trust what you have built.

Solo: record yourself play back + self-audit	**Paired: actor has all info** candidate sees brief only	**Blank? Use ICE** always safe recovery	**Error? Correct aloud** honesty scores marks	**Unwell patient: STOP** ABCDE immediately
Run out of time close + safety-net first	**Bad station: reset** 3 breaths + new brief	**Day 7: no new content** trust what you have built	**Model performance** calibration not memorisation	**Self-audit after each** unticked = drill needed

Model Performances — All 18 Stations

Each performance shows a top-scoring candidate. Bold phrases score marks. Italic actions are examiner-visible. CAUTION — marks an instant-fail risk moment.

Use these to calibrate your rehearsal — not to memorise verbatim. The benchmark matters; the exact wording does not.

STATION 1

ACUTE CHEST PAIN (Possible ACS)

Model Performance · Self-Audit Checklist · 8 Minutes

Model Performance — Top-Scoring Candidate

SAY — Bold = mark-scoring phrases · *Italic = examiner-visible actions* · **CAUTION — = instant-fail risk moment**

0:00–0:30	**Enter + Assess**	*Knock, enter. Eye contact. Wash hands visibly. Scan patient — diaphoretic, clutching chest.* **"Hello, I'm Dr Mansour, one of the doctors. Can I confirm your name and date of birth? Thank you, Mr James."** **"I can see you're in pain right now — I want to help you quickly. I'm going to check your vital signs while we talk — is that okay?"** *Apply SpO_2 probe, attach cardiac monitor, note HR/BP.* **Do NOT give oxygen yet — check SpO_2 first.**

0:30–2:30	**ABCDE + History**	**"Airway — you're speaking so airway is clear. Breathing — RR normal, SpO_2 97% on air — no oxygen needed. Circulation — HR 98, BP 144/88. Getting IV access and requesting urgent ECG now."** *Call nurse: "Urgent ECG in the next five minutes please — possible ACS."* **"Tell me about the pain. Where exactly? Does it go anywhere — your arm, jaw, back?"** **"On a scale of 0 to 10, how severe? When exactly did it start? Anything like this before?"** **"Any sweating, nausea, shortness of breath?"** **"What do you think might be happening? What worries you most right now?"**
2:30–4:30	**ECG + Management**	*ECG reviewed: ST elevation II, III, aVF.* **"The ECG shows changes I'm very concerned about — this looks like a heart attack. Specifically, this is an inferior STEMI."** **Before aspirin: "Do you have any allergies, especially to aspirin or NSAIDs?"** **"No allergies — I'm giving you aspirin 300mg to chew now. This helps prevent further clotting."** **"I'm escalating immediately to the cardiology team for primary PCI."** *"This is Dr Mansour, FY2 in ED. 55-year-old male, inferior STEMI, onset 45 minutes, haemodynamically stable. Requesting immediate cardiology review for primary PCI."*
4:30–7:00	**Explain + ICE**	**"Mr James, I want to explain clearly. You are having a heart attack. This is serious but you're in exactly the right place."** **"The cardiology team is coming to take you for a procedure to open the blocked artery. The sooner we do this, the better."** **"I know this is frightening. That's completely understandable. Is there anyone you'd like us to contact?"** *Document time zero, ECG time, aspirin time, cardiology call time.*
7:00–8:00	**Close + Safety-net**	**"To summarise — you are having an inferior heart attack. Aspirin given. Cardiology on their way. You are monitored continuously."** **"If your pain worsens, if you feel faint, or anything changes — tell the nursing team immediately. You will not be left alone."** **"Do you have any questions before I hand you over to the cardiology team?"** *Document: time zero, ECG findings, aspirin given, SBAR, monitoring in progress.*

Station 1 — Self-Audit (10 points)

After your practice run, tick each item honestly. Any unticked = targeted drill needed.

#	Did you...	✓/X
1	Introduce + confirm patient ID in first 20 seconds	

#	Did you...	✓/X
2	Attach monitoring (SpO_2/cardiac) before or during history	
3	Characterise pain using SOCRATES systematically	
4	Ask specifically about radiation (jaw/arm), sweating, nausea	
5	Request ECG within 10 minutes of presentation	
6	Check SpO_2 before prescribing oxygen (only if <94%)	
7	Prescribe aspirin 300mg AFTER allergy check	
8	Escalate to cardiology with SBAR urgency language	
9	Acknowledge patient distress with empathy phrase	
10	Deliver safety-net before closing station	

STATION 2

PAEDIATRIC FEVER & BREATHING DIFFICULTY

Model Performance · Self-Audit Checklist · 8 Minutes

Model Performance — Top-Scoring Candidate

SAY — Bold = mark-scoring phrases · *Italic = examiner-visible actions* · **CAUTION — = instant-fail risk moment**

0:00–0:30	Assess + ABC	*Enter. Scan child: respiratory effort, colour, alertness. SpO_2 probe immediately.* **"Hello, I'm Dr Mansour. You must be Mrs Thomas — and this is Tommy. I can see he's working harder to breathe. I'm assessing him right away."** **"SpO_2 is 95%, RR is 42 — elevated. I can see nasal flaring and mild recession. I'm starting oxygen via nasal cannula now while we talk."**
0:30–2:30	Focused History	**"How long has the fever been? Have you measured his temperature? What have you given to bring it down?"** **"How is his feeding? Roughly what percentage of his normal feed has he taken today?"** **Critical trigger — ask directly: "Is he taking his normal amount or less?"** **"Has he had any wet nappies today? Any rash? Any seizures or floppy episodes?"** **"Was he born at full term? Any previous admissions?"** **"What was your main concern when you brought him in today?"**

2:30–5:00	**Explain + Management**	**"Tommy has a fever and his breathing is faster than normal. In a child his age, this is likely a viral infection affecting his airways — something called bronchiolitis or a chest infection."** **"His oxygen is borderline at 95%. I'm going to escalate to the paediatric team for urgent review."** **"I can see this is really worrying. You were absolutely right to bring him in."**
5:00–8:00	**Safety-net + Close**	**"While we wait for the paediatric team: if Tommy becomes difficult to rouse, if his lips go blue, if he has a seizure, or his breathing becomes much more laboured — call us immediately."** **"Any questions for me?"** *Document: temp, SpO_2, RR, feeding %, escalation, oxygen started, safety-net given.*

Station 2 — Self-Audit (10 points)

After your practice run, tick each item honestly. Any unticked = targeted drill needed.

#	Did you…	✓/✗
1	Address parent by name and introduce yourself clearly	
2	Assess SpO_2 and work of breathing within first minute	
3	Ask specifically about feeding volume (how much vs normal)	
4	Ask about rash, seizures, fontanelle, neck stiffness	
5	Ask about wet nappies/urine output in last 12 hours	
6	Give oxygen if SpO_2 <92% without delay	
7	Use NICE traffic light to classify (red/amber/green)	
8	Apply SAFE-D: SpO_2 + Work of Breathing + Fever + Escalation + Dehydration	
9	Deliver clear safety-net with specific red flags for parent	
10	Escalate — paediatric review if any red flags present	

SAY — STATION 3

BREAKING BAD NEWS (SPIKES + NURSE)

Model Performance · Self-Audit Checklist · 8 Minutes

Model Performance — Top-Scoring Candidate

SAY — Bold = mark-scoring phrases · *Italic = examiner-visible actions* · **CAUTION — = instant-fail risk moment**

0:00–0:45	SPIKES S + P	*Private room, tissues visible, sit at patient level.* **"Hello Mrs Ahmed, I'm Dr Mansour. Before we begin, I want to make sure we have enough time together. Is it alright if we talk here?"** **"I'd like to start by checking in with you. What have you been told about why you're here today?"** **"And in your own mind — what were you thinking might be going on?"** *Listen carefully. Let her speak. This reveals how much she knows.*
0:45–2:00	SPIKES I + K	**"The results are back from the biopsy and I have some news to share. Before I tell you — are you happy for me to go through the results now?"** **"I'm afraid the news I have to share is not what we were hoping for." (Warning shot. Pause. Wait for response.)** **"The biopsy has confirmed that this is cancer — a type called invasive ductal carcinoma of the breast."** *STOP. Put down any paper. Full eye contact. Complete silence. Wait.* **Do NOT continue speaking. The pause is the most important moment in this station.**
2:00–4:30	NURSE Empathy	*Patient may cry. Move slightly forward. Offer tissues. Stay silent until she is ready.* **"I can only imagine how frightening that word sounds." (Name the emotion)** **"It's completely understandable to feel overwhelmed right now." (Understand)** **"I'm here with you, and we are going to go through every step of this together." (Support)** **"Can I ask — what is going through your mind right now?" (Explore)**
4:30–6:30	Clinical Plan	**"When you feel ready, I'd like to explain what happens next — only when you're ready."** **"This type of cancer is treatable. You'll be referred to a specialist breast cancer team who will create a plan specifically for you."** **Do NOT give survival statistics unless directly asked.** **"You will have a breast cancer nurse specialist assigned to you — she will be your main point of contact throughout."**
6:30–8:00	Close + Written Info	**"I'd like to give you some written information to take home."** **"Is there someone you'd like us to contact, or who you'd like to have with you?"** **"If anything comes up before your next appointment — any questions, any concerns — please call us. You do not need to wait."** *Document: results explained, patient understanding, emotional response, support offered, follow-up arranged.*

Station 3 — Self-Audit (10 points)

After your practice run, tick each item honestly. Any unticked = targeted drill needed.

#	Did you...	✓/X
1	Confirm private setting before starting	
2	SPIKES: Setting → Perception → Invitation → Knowledge → Empathy → Strategy	
3	Fire a warning shot before delivering the diagnosis	
4	Check perception first: "What have you been told / what do you think?"	
5	Say the word "cancer" clearly — no euphemisms	
6	PAUSE after delivering the diagnosis — allow silence	
7	NURSE: Name / Understand / Respect / Support / Explore	
8	Do NOT continue with clinical information while patient is crying	
9	Offer written information and cancer support helpline	
10	Do NOT give unsolicited prognosis statistics	

STATION 4

CAPACITY ASSESSMENT (Refusing Insulin)

Model Performance · Self-Audit Checklist · 8 Minutes

Model Performance — Top-Scoring Candidate

SAY — **Bold = mark-scoring phrases** · *Italic = examiner-visible actions* · **CAUTION — = instant-fail risk moment**

0:00–1:00	**Rapport + Stage 1**	**"Hello Mr Jones, I'm Dr Mansour. Thank you for speaking with me. I understand you have concerns about the insulin — I want to understand your thinking before we discuss anything further."** **"First — how are you feeling generally today? Any pain, any confusion?"** *Oriented, coherent, appropriate = no obvious impairment.* **"Your blood glucose is 24 — that's quite high and I do need to discuss this with you. But first I want to hear your concerns."**

1:00–3:30	**URWC Assessment**	**"Can you tell me in your own words what you understand about why we're recommending insulin today?" (Understand)** **"If you decided not to have it — what do you think could happen?" (Weigh up)** **"You mentioned earlier you had a bad experience. Can you tell me what happened?" (Hidden info trigger — explore hypo fear)** **"That sounds absolutely frightening — collapsing like that. I completely understand why that would make you cautious about insulin." (Empathy before clinical argument)** **"Can you tell me what your decision is, and why?" (Communicate)**

3:30–5:30	**Risk + Alternatives**	**"I want to be honest with you. A blood glucose of 24 means your body is in a dangerous state. Without insulin there is a real risk of DKA — diabetic ketoacidosis — which can cause unconsciousness."** **Do NOT say: "If you don't have the insulin you could die." This is coercive.** **"I want to address your hypoglycaemia fear directly. If you agree to insulin today, I want to monitor you very closely and explain exactly what to look for."** **"Could we start on a very low dose with close monitoring? What do you think?"**

5:30–8:00	**Document + Escalate**	**"Mr Jones, based on our conversation, I believe you have the capacity to make this decision. You have understood the risks, weighed them up, and communicated a clear choice."** **"I'm going to document this carefully — your decision, your reasons, the risks I've explained. I also need to involve my senior."** *Document: assessment performed, capacity present, limbs tested, conclusion, plan, senior informed.*

Station 4 — Self-Audit (10 points)

After your practice run, tick each item honestly. Any unticked = targeted drill needed.

#	Did you...	✓/X
1	Introduce and build rapport BEFORE beginning assessment	
2	Stage 1: identify the impairment — assess this first	
3	URWC: Understand / Retain / Weigh up / Communicate	
4	Ask open questions to test each limb — do not lead	
5	Explore the REASON for refusal (hidden: hypo fear)	
6	Explain DKA risk clearly in plain language	

#	Did you...	✓/X
7	Capacity PRESENT: respect decision + document + alternatives + senior	
8	NEVER coerce, threaten, or pressure in any way	
9	Offer alternatives that address the patient's specific concern	
10	Document: assessment performed, conclusion, reasoning, plan	

STATION 5

INPATIENT DRUG CHART (CAP, Penicillin Allergy)

Model Performance · Self-Audit Checklist · 8 Minutes

Model Performance — Top-Scoring Candidate

SAY — Bold = mark-scoring phrases · *Italic = examiner-visible actions* · **CAUTION — = instant-fail risk moment**

0:00–1:00	**Allergy Check First**	**"Hello Mr Brown, I'm Dr Mansour. Before I do anything else — do you have any allergies to medications?"** **"You mentioned penicillin — what exactly happened? Was it a skin rash? Any swelling of your face or lips? Any breathing difficulty?"** *Hidden info: rash only, no anaphylaxis.* **"Thank you — so a skin rash but no breathing difficulty. That's important because it changes which antibiotics are safe for you. I'm documenting this now in red — penicillin, reaction: rash only."** **If anaphylaxis: all beta-lactams must be avoided. Rash = lower cross-reactivity risk.**
1:00–3:00	**Clinical Reasoning**	**"Let me explain what I'm treating and why I'm choosing a particular antibiotic."** **"You have community-acquired pneumonia. Your CURB-65 score is 2 — moderately unwell, needs antibiotics with close monitoring."** **"Because of your penicillin allergy I cannot use amoxicillin. Instead I'm prescribing doxycycline — the recommended alternative."** **"Your creatinine is 140 — slightly above normal. Doxycycline is safe at normal doses with this level but I'm documenting it for review."**
3:00–5:30	**Prescribe + Counsel**	*Prescribe: Doxycycline 200mg loading dose then 100mg OD for 5 days. Sign, date, indication, allergy noted.* **"I'm prescribing doxycycline. First dose is slightly larger. Then one tablet daily for five days."** **"Take it with a full glass of water and stay upright for 30 minutes — it can cause heartburn if you lie down. Take with food if it upsets your stomach."** **"I'll review you in 48 hours. If you're not improving or feel worse — let the nursing staff know immediately."**

5:30–8:00	Safety-net + Close	**"Important: if you develop any new rash, swelling of your lips or throat, or any difficulty breathing — press the call bell immediately."** **"Any questions about the antibiotic or what to expect?"** *Document: allergy documented, antibiotic rationale, duration, review plan, patient counselled.*

Station 5 — Self-Audit (10 points)

After your practice run, tick each item honestly. Any unticked = targeted drill needed.

#	Did you...	✓/X
1	Ask about allergy FIRST — before any prescribing	
2	Characterise the reaction: rash (low risk) vs anaphylaxis (high risk)	
3	Document allergy in red on drug chart with reaction type	
4	Choose correct antibiotic (doxycycline or clarithromycin for pen allergy + CAP)	
5	Consider renal function — creatinine 140 requires documentation	
6	Apply CURB-65 = 2 to determine route and duration (5 days)	
7	Explain antibiotic choice to patient in plain language	
8	Arrange 48-hour review and state duration clearly	
9	Use ACID-ID checklist before prescribing	
10	Safety-net: rash worsens, breathing difficulty → seek help immediately	

THINK — STATION 6

ACUTE STROKE (Time-Critical Thrombolysis)

Model Performance · Self-Audit Checklist · 8 Minutes

Model Performance — Top-Scoring Candidate

SAY — Bold = mark-scoring phrases · *Italic = examiner-visible actions* · **CAUTION — = instant-fail risk moment**

0:00–0:45	FAST + TIME ZERO	*Enter urgently. Patient right arm limp, dysarthric. Wife at bedside.* **"FAST: Face — asymmetry present. Arms — right arm drifting. Speech — slurred. Time — Mrs Khan, when exactly did this start? Three hours ago confirmed."** **"Blood glucose checking now — 5.8, normal. Not a hypoglycaemic episode."** **"I'm calling the stroke team now." Call: "Suspected stroke, FAST positive, onset 3 hours, within thrombolysis window. Urgent stroke team review."**

0:45–2:30	**Assessment + CT**	**"Ordering urgent CT head now — to look at the brain and decide on treatment."** **"BP 176/102, HR 88 irregular — AF. I need to check INR urgently. Is Mr Khan on any blood thinners?"** Do NOT give aspirin until CT is back. **"Mrs Khan — your husband may be having a stroke. We are treating this as an emergency. There is a treatment we may be able to give, but we need the scan first."**

2:30–8:00	**CT + Decision + Family**	*CT result: no haemorrhage. INR 1.2.* **"No bleeding on CT — good news. Handing over to stroke consultant for thrombolysis decision."** **"SBAR: Mr Khan, 67. Suspected left MCA stroke, FAST positive, onset 3 hours, BG 5.8, AF, INR 1.2, no haemorrhage on CT. For thrombolysis consideration."** **"Mrs Khan — we are acting as quickly as possible. Time is critical. Is there anything you want to ask me?"** *Document: FAST time, BG, CT time, INR, stroke team, aspirin withheld, SBAR recorded.*

Station 6 — Self-Audit (10 points)

After your practice run, tick each item honestly. Any unticked = targeted drill needed.

#	Did you…	✓/✗
1	FAST immediately: Face / Arms / Speech / Time of onset	
2	Document exact time of onset (4.5-hour window for thrombolysis)	
3	Check blood glucose immediately (exclude hypoglycaemia mimic)	
4	Call stroke team immediately — do not wait for CT	
5	Order urgent non-contrast CT head	
6	Do NOT give aspirin until CT excludes haemorrhage	
7	Check INR/anticoagulants (warfarin = contraindication risk)	
8	Communicate urgency without causing panic	
9	Explain thrombolysis if CT confirms ischaemic + no contraindications	
10	Document: FAST, time, BG, BP, AF, escalation time	

STATION 7

ANAPHYLAXIS (RCUK Algorithm)

Model Performance · Self-Audit Checklist · 8 Minutes

Model Performance — Top-Scoring Candidate

SAY — Bold = mark-scoring phrases · *Italic = examiner-visible actions* · **CAUTION — = instant-fail risk moment**

0:00–0:30	**Recognise + Call**	*Enter. Ms Patel: flushed, swollen lips, audible wheeze, scratching arms.* **"Ms Patel, I can see you're having a serious allergic reaction. I'm calling for help right now."** *"I need IMMEDIATE help — suspected anaphylaxis. Emergency trolley, adrenaline, second person NOW."* **"I'm going to give you an injection right now. It's adrenaline — it will help immediately."**

0:30–2:00	**AIR Protocol**	**Adrenaline FIRST. Before antihistamines. Before steroids. Before anything else.** **"IM adrenaline 0.5mg from the 1:1000 solution — into the anterolateral thigh. Given now."** *Draw up 0.5mL from 1:1000. IM injection anterolateral thigh. Document time.* **"High-flow oxygen — 15 litres via non-rebreather mask. Sitting her up as she's having breathing difficulty."** **"IV access — two large-bore cannulae. 500mL crystalloid if BP drops."** **"If she's not improving in 5 minutes, I'll repeat the IM adrenaline. Routine antihistamines and steroids are no longer recommended in acute anaphylaxis — a non-sedating oral antihistamine can come later if she has skin symptoms once stable."**

2:00–8:00	**Monitor + Plan**	**"Ms Patel, the adrenaline should start helping in the next few minutes. Can you tell me — did you eat anything before this happened? Did it contain nuts or sesame?"** **"Mast cell tryptase needed now, at 1 hour, and 24 hours — requesting from lab."** **"You're looking better. SpO_2 back to 98%, wheeze improved. Monitoring for biphasic reaction — risk-stratified, 6–12 hours."** **"Before you go home — I'm prescribing you an Epipen and teaching you how to use it. Allergy clinic referral arranged."** *Document: adrenaline dose + time, response, tryptase times, Epipen prescribed, allergy referral.*

Station 7 — Self-Audit (10 points)

After your practice run, tick each item honestly. Any unticked = targeted drill needed.

#	Did you...	✓/X
1	Recognise: urticaria + wheeze/stridor + hypotension after allergen	
2	Call for help SIMULTANEOUSLY — do not delay adrenaline	
3	IM adrenaline 0.5mg (1:1000) anterolateral thigh — FIRST action	
4	Correct concentration: 1:1000 NOT 1:10,000	
5	Position: sit up if breathing difficulty, lie flat if hypotensive	

#	Did you...	✓/X
6	High-flow oxygen 15L via non-rebreather mask	
7	IV access + 500mL crystalloid if hypotensive	
8	Repeat IM adrenaline at 5 min if no response; recognise refractory anaphylaxis (RCUK 2021: no routine antihistamine/steroid)	
9	Monitor for biphasic reaction — observe, risk-stratified 6–12 hours (longer if severe/refractory)	
10	Identify trigger, allergy clinic referral, prescribe Epipen on discharge	

STATION 8

SEPSIS (Sepsis-6 within 1 Hour)

Model Performance · Self-Audit Checklist · 8 Minutes

Model Performance — Top-Scoring Candidate

SAY — Bold = mark-scoring phrases · *Italic = examiner-visible actions* · **CAUTION — = instant-fail risk moment**

0:00–0:45	**Recognise + TIME ZERO**	*Enter. Mrs White: confused, shivering, pale. HR 118, BP 88/52, RR 28, Temp 38.9.* **"I'm Dr Mansour. Mrs White, can you hear me? I'm going to help you."** **"Calling for immediate help. This patient has suspected sepsis. TIME ZERO is now — documenting the time."** **"NEWS2: HR 118, BP 88/52, RR 28, SpO_2 91%, Temp 38.9, confused. High score — this is a medical emergency."**

0:45–2:30	**Sepsis-6: TAKE**	**"TAKE blood cultures first — two sets from two sites BEFORE antibiotics."** **"TAKE lactate — requesting VBG urgently."** **"TAKE urine output — catheter in situ, connecting to bag. Urine output 15mL in last 2 hours — critically low."** *Hidden info: lactate 4.2, catheter 8 days.* **"Lactate is 4.2 mmol/L. This is septic shock. I need ICU review immediately."**

2:30–4:30	**Sepsis-6: GIVE**	**"GIVE oxygen — 15L via non-rebreather mask."** **"GIVE IV antibiotics within 1 hour of time zero. Blood cultures taken. Giving piperacillin-tazobactam now — broad spectrum, covers urinary source."** **"GIVE IV fluids — 500mL crystalloid bolus. Reassessing BP and urine output after."** **"SBAR to ICU: Mrs White, 71, septic shock, catheter UTI source, lactate 4.2, BP 88/52. Sepsis-6 in progress. Requesting ICU review."**

4:30–8:00	Reassess + Document	*After bolus: BP 96/60, HR 108 — slight improvement.* **"BP slightly improved. Still tachycardic, urine output low. Continuing Sepsis-6, considering second bolus."** **"Catheter in situ 8 days — discussing source removal with the team."** *Document: time zero, all 6 Sepsis-6 actions with times, lactate, escalation, antibiotic, urine output trend.*

Station 8 — Self-Audit (10 points)

After your practice run, tick each item honestly. Any unticked = targeted drill needed.

#	Did you...	✓/X
1	Recognise: infection + organ dysfunction + haemodynamic compromise	
2	Document TIME ZERO immediately	
3	Blood cultures ×2 BEFORE antibiotics	
4	Lactate/VBG — >4 = septic shock	
5	Catheterise and monitor urine output	
6	IV antibiotics within 1 hour of TIME ZERO	
7	500mL crystalloid bolus if lactate elevated or hypotensive	
8	Oxygen — target SpO_2 ≥94%	
9	Escalate immediately — ICU if lactate >4	
10	SBAR to handover: source, NEWS2, lactate, time zero, Sepsis-6 status	

STATION 9

PAEDIATRIC BRONCHIOLITIS (NICE NG9)

Model Performance · Self-Audit Checklist · 8 Minutes

Model Performance — Top-Scoring Candidate

SAY — **Bold = mark-scoring phrases** · *Italic = examiner-visible actions* · CAUTION — = instant-fail risk moment

0:00–0:30	Assess + ABC	*Enter. Scan baby: tachypnoeic, nasal flaring, mild recession. SpO_2 91%.* **"Hello, I'm Dr Mansour. You must be Mr and Mrs Singh. I can see Priya is working harder to breathe. I'm assessing her right away."** **"SpO_2 is 91% — lower than we'd like. RR 58 — elevated. Nasal flaring and mild recession. I'm starting oxygen via nasal cannula right now."**

0:30–2:30	Focused History	"How long has she been unwell? How did it start?" "How is her feeding? Roughly what percentage of her normal feed has she had today?" Critical trigger — ask directly about feeding amount. "Has she had any episodes where she seemed to stop breathing or go very pale?" Critical trigger: apnoea at home. Ask directly. "Was she born at full term? Any complications at birth?"

2:30–5:00	Explain + Plan	"Priya has bronchiolitis — a viral infection causing inflammation in the small airways. Very common in babies under 2." "Because of three things — low oxygen, reduced feeding, and the brief episode at home where she seemed to stop breathing — I want to admit Priya for monitoring tonight." NICE NG9: NO routine suctioning. NO salbutamol. NO steroids. "The treatment for bronchiolitis is supportive: oxygen, feeding support, monitoring. We do not use inhalers or steroids for this — the evidence does not support them and they can cause harm."

5:00–8:00	Safety-net + Close	"If Priya is not taking 50% of her normal feed, we'll use a small nasal feeding tube so she gets nutrition without exhausting herself." "What worries you most right now?" (ICE) "You both did exactly the right thing bringing her in today." *Document: SpO_2, RR, feeding %, apnoea, prematurity, admission plan, oxygen started, salbutamol/steroids withheld with reason.*

Station 9 — Self-Audit (10 points)

After your practice run, tick each item honestly. Any unticked = targeted drill needed.

#	Did you...	✓/X
1	Introduce to both parents, acknowledge baby	
2	Assess SpO_2 and work of breathing immediately	
3	Ask specifically about feeding volume (hidden: 30% of normal)	
4	Ask about apnoea at home (hidden: yes — high risk)	
5	Note prematurity (hidden: 34 weeks — higher risk)	
6	Oxygen via nasal cannula if SpO_2 <92%	
7	NG feeding if <50% volume or fatiguing	
8	Do NOT perform routine nasopharyngeal suctioning (NICE NG9)	
9	Do NOT prescribe salbutamol or steroids (NICE NG9)	
10	Admit for monitoring — explain rationale honestly	

STATION 10

POSTPARTUM HAEMORRHAGE (PPH)

Model Performance · Self-Audit Checklist · 8 Minutes

Model Performance — Top-Scoring Candidate

SAY — Bold = mark-scoring phrases · *Italic = examiner-visible actions* · **CAUTION — = instant-fail risk moment**

0:00–0:30	**Call + Two IVs**	**"CALL FOR HELP NOW. Senior obstetrician, anaesthetist, midwife at bedside. PPH."** *Two large-bore IV cannulae. Bloods: FBC, clotting, X-match 4 units, fibrinogen.* **"Mrs Green, I'm Dr Mansour. You're losing more blood than normal after delivery. We're treating this right now — I have a team here."** **"I'm catheterising your bladder now — a full bladder stops the uterus contracting properly."**
0:30–2:30	**4 Ts + Oxytocin**	**"4 Ts: Tone — uterus boggy, atony most likely. Trauma — checking for lacerations. Tissue — placenta delivered intact. Thrombin — clotting screen sent."** **"Bimanual uterine massage now. Oxytocin 10 units IM given — or 5 units by slow IV injection. Tranexamic acid 1g IV over 10 minutes, given early. Senior obstetric team for further uterotonics (ergometrine/carboprost) if bleeding continues."** **"500mL crystalloid bolus running. EBL now 1100mL and ongoing."** **If EBL ≥1500mL: activate major haemorrhage protocol.**
2:30–8:00	**Escalate + Support**	**"Activating major haemorrhage protocol — EBL 1500mL. Blood products on their way."** **"Mr Green — your wife is losing more blood than normal after delivery. We are treating this as an emergency and we have a full team here. She is in the right place."** *Document: time, EBL estimates, interventions with times, medications, blood products, escalation.*

Station 10 — Self-Audit (10 points)

After your practice run, tick each item honestly. Any unticked = targeted drill needed.

#	Did you...	✓/✗
1	Call for help immediately: senior obs + anaesthetist + midwife	
2	Two large-bore IV cannulae + FBC/clotting/X-match 4 units	
3	Catheterise bladder (full bladder prevents uterine contraction)	
4	Bimanual uterine massage + fundal assessment	

#	Did you...	✓/✗
5	Oxytocin 10 units IM, or 5 units by slow IV injection (not 10 IV); tranexamic acid 1g IV early	
6	4 Ts: Tone / Trauma / Tissue / Thrombin	
7	Cross-match + activate major haemorrhage protocol if >1500mL	
8	Document blood loss, all interventions with times	
9	Communicate calmly to patient and partner despite urgency	
10	Escalate to senior if no response to oxytocin within 15 minutes	

STATION 11

REDUCED FETAL MOVEMENTS

Model Performance · Self-Audit Checklist · 8 Minutes

Model Performance — Top-Scoring Candidate

SAY — Bold = mark-scoring phrases · *Italic = examiner-visible actions* · **CAUTION — = instant-fail risk moment**

0:00–1:30	**History + CTG**	**"Hello Mrs Clarke, I'm Dr Mansour. You've noticed reduced movements. When did you first notice this?"** **Critical: "Has it just been today, or has it been longer than that?"** **"And normally — how often does the baby move? Does the baby have a pattern you recognise?"** **"I want to start monitoring the baby's heartbeat while we talk. I'm requesting a CTG right now."**
1:30–4:00	**Full History + Plan**	**"Any bleeding? Pain? Headaches or visual changes? Swelling of hands or face?"** **"How has your pregnancy been overall? Any concerns at scans?"** **"I want to be honest with you. The fact that movements have reduced for three days — not just today — means we need to investigate this properly."** **"In addition to the CTG I'd like to arrange an ultrasound scan today to check baby's growth and fluid levels."**
4:00–8:00	**CTG Result + Communicate**	**"The CTG shows: baseline 150, reduced variability, no accelerations. This pattern needs further assessment."** **Do NOT say "I'm sure everything is fine."** **"I want to be honest — the CTG isn't showing the pattern we'd ideally like to see. I'm involving the senior midwife and obstetric consultant."** **"You were absolutely right to come in. Going forward: if movements stop or you feel something is wrong — do not wait. Come in immediately."**

Station 11 — Self-Audit (10 points)

After your practice run, tick each item honestly. Any unticked = targeted drill needed.

#	Did you...	✓/X
1	Establish how long movements reduced (hidden: 3 days not just today)	
2	Ask about normal movement pattern for this baby	
3	Assess for risk factors: reduced liquor, IUGR, placental insufficiency	
4	Do NOT reassure without investigations — this is a fail trigger	
5	Order CTG immediately — do not wait for full history	
6	Request ultrasound if CTG reassuring (growth, liquor, Doppler)	
7	Explain CTG findings honestly	
8	Do not use "I'm sure everything is fine" — false reassurance	
9	Safety-net: any decrease in movements → come back immediately	
10	Document: duration reduced movements, CTG result, plan	

THINK — STATION 12

SELF-HARM RISK ASSESSMENT

Model Performance · Self-Audit Checklist · 8 Minutes

Model Performance — Top-Scoring Candidate

SAY — **Bold = mark-scoring phrases** · *Italic = examiner-visible actions* · **CAUTION — = instant-fail risk moment**

0:00–1:30	**Rapport First**	*Wounds dressed. Room private. Sit at same level. Unhurried posture.* **"Hello Sam. I'm Dr Mansour. I'm really glad you're here today. Before we talk about anything medical — how are you feeling right now?"** **"There's no rush. I'm not going anywhere."** **"I know it might feel difficult to talk. You don't have to share anything you're not ready to share. But I want to understand what's been happening for you."**
1:30–4:00	**Context + RASSO**	**"Can you tell me a bit about what's been going on in your life recently? What has today been like for you?"** **"The cuts on your arms — can you help me understand what was happening for you when that occurred?"** **"I need to ask you directly — asking this is important and will not make things worse: were you thinking about ending your life?"** **"Do you have thoughts like that now? Do you have a plan?"** **"What has helped you get through difficult times before? Is there anyone you trust?"**

4:00–8:00	Safety Plan + Team	**"Thank you for telling me all of this, Sam. I take what you've shared seriously."** **"I'd like you to speak with the psychiatric liaison team today — they specialise in exactly this kind of support."** **"Before you leave, I want to make a plan with you. If the urge to hurt yourself comes back, what could you do? Is there someone you could call?"** **"We won't discharge you today without a proper plan in place."** *Document: risk assessment, ideation/plan/intent, protective factors, psychiatric review arranged, safety plan.*

Station 12 — Self-Audit (10 points)

After your practice run, tick each item honestly. Any unticked = targeted drill needed.

#	Did you...	✓/X
1	Physical safety first: wounds dressed, vitals stable	
2	Establish privacy before beginning any risk assessment	
3	Build therapeutic rapport BEFORE asking about self-harm details	
4	Explore context and emotional state before intent/plan questions	
5	Ask directly about suicidal intent — this does NOT plant the idea	
6	RASSO: Reason / Access / Severity / Supports / Other harm	
7	Identify protective factors: reasons to live, future plans, support	
8	Do NOT discharge without psychiatric review or crisis plan	
9	Involve psychiatric liaison or mental health team	
10	Safety plan: what Sam will do if urge to self-harm returns	

STATION 13

ALCOHOL WITHDRAWAL (CIWA-Ar)

Model Performance · Self-Audit Checklist · 8 Minutes

Model Performance — Top-Scoring Candidate

SAY — Bold = mark-scoring phrases · *Italic = examiner-visible actions* · **CAUTION — = instant-fail risk moment**

0:00–1:00	Recognise + Thiamine FIRST	*Enter. Mr Hughes: sweating, tremulous, anxious. HR 112, BP 152/96.* **"Mr Hughes, I'm Dr Mansour. I can see you're very uncomfortable. I want to help you."** **Do NOT give glucose yet.** **"Before anything else, I'm giving you IV Pabrinex — thiamine. I need to give this before any glucose because without it, glucose can cause serious brain damage."** **"IV Pabrinex given. Blood glucose: 3.8. Glucose replacement can now safely follow."**

1:00–3:30	CIWA + History	**"I'm going to ask you about some symptoms. This helps me understand how severe the withdrawal is."** **"Nausea? Sweating? Tremor? Anxiety? Any unusual sounds or visions?"** **"When did you last have a drink? And roughly how much do you drink on a typical day?"** **Hidden info trigger: ask directly about daily amount.** **"Have you ever had a seizure during withdrawal? Or confusion or hallucinations this severe before?"**

3:30–8:00	Treatment + Escalate	**"CIWA score approximately 14 — moderate severity. I'm starting symptom-triggered chlordiazepoxide to prevent seizures and manage the withdrawal."** **"I'm monitoring your vital signs continuously. If your confusion worsens or you develop hallucinations — I'm escalating to my senior immediately."** **"I want to talk about your drinking when you're feeling better — before you leave hospital. There is real support available."** *Document: CIWA score, thiamine before glucose, chlordiazepoxide regime, vital signs, escalation plan.*

Station 13 — Self-Audit (10 points)

After your practice run, tick each item honestly. Any unticked = targeted drill needed.

#	Did you…	✓/X
1	Identify withdrawal: sweating, tremor, agitation after last drink (36 hours)	
2	CIWA-Ar: 10 domains including tremor, sweating, anxiety, nausea, perceptual disturbances	
3	Give IV Pabrinex (thiamine) BEFORE glucose — prevents Wernicke's encephalopathy	
4	Ask specifically about daily intake (hidden: 15–20 units/day for 5 years)	
5	Ask about previous withdrawal complications: seizures, delirium tremens	
6	Chlordiazepoxide or lorazepam for symptom-triggered protocol	
7	Monitor vitals: HR, BP, temperature — autonomic instability risk	
8	Check glucose (hypoglycaemia common in alcohol misuse)	

#	Did you…	✓/X
9	MUST NOT give glucose BEFORE thiamine — critical fail trigger	
10	Escalate if CIWA >15 or signs of delirium tremens	

STATION 14

CONSENT FOR LUMBAR PUNCTURE

Model Performance · Self-Audit Checklist · 8 Minutes

Model Performance — Top-Scoring Candidate

SAY — **Bold = mark-scoring phrases** · *Italic = examiner-visible actions* · CAUTION — = instant-fail risk moment

0:00–1:30	Indication + ICE	**"Hello Mr Shah, I'm Dr Mansour. I'd like to explain a procedure we'd like to do today. Before I explain it — what have you been told about why we want to do this?"** **"We'd like to do a lumbar puncture. The reason is to look at the fluid around your brain and spinal cord. Given your severe headache, neck stiffness, and light sensitivity, we need to make sure there's no serious infection or bleeding that the CT scan couldn't fully rule out."**
1:30–4:00	Procedure + Risks	**"You'll be asked to curl into a ball on your side. We clean the skin in the lower back, inject local anaesthetic so the area goes numb, then pass a thin needle between two vertebrae to collect a small amount of fluid."** **"The most common side effect is a headache afterwards — this happens in about 1 in 3 people. Manageable with rest and fluids."** **"Rare but more serious: bleeding, infection, or nerve irritation. Paralysis is extremely rare with a properly performed LP."** Hidden info trigger: "Is there anything specifically worrying you about this procedure?" **"A lumbar puncture is different from an epidural. An epidural delivers medication through a catheter. An LP is a single brief procedure with a much finer needle. The chronic back pain risk is much lower."**
4:00–8:00	Questions + Consent	**"Do you have any other concerns I haven't addressed?"** **"This is your choice. I'm recommending it because it could give vital information. But if you decide you don't want it, I will respect that."** **"If you're happy to go ahead, I'll ask you to sign a consent form. I can also give you a written leaflet."** *Document: indication explained, all material risks discussed, understanding confirmed, consent given/refused.*

Station 14 — Self-Audit (10 points)

After your practice run, tick each item honestly. Any unticked = targeted drill needed.

#	Did you...	✓/X
1	Introduce and confirm capacity before discussing procedure	
2	Explain INDICATION clearly: exclude bacterial meningitis / SAH	
3	Describe procedure step-by-step in plain language	
4	Most common risk: post-LP headache (1 in 3) — must be mentioned	
5	Serious but rare: nerve damage, bleeding, infection	
6	Address patient's specific concern (hidden: friend with chronic back pain after epidural)	
7	Explain LP is different from epidural — address directly	
8	If refuses: respect, explore, document, offer alternatives	
9	Do NOT pressure or rush — consent must be voluntary	
10	Offer written information leaflet	

STATION 15

INSULIN PRESCRIPTION (VRIII)

Model Performance · Self-Audit Checklist · 8 Minutes

Model Performance — Top-Scoring Candidate

SAY — **Bold = mark-scoring phrases** · *Italic = examiner-visible actions* · **CAUTION — = instant-fail risk moment**

0:00–1:30	**Diabetes History**	**"Hello Mrs Okafor, I'm Dr Mansour. I'm here to talk about your diabetes and surgery tomorrow."** **"Tell me about your diabetes — how long? How is it controlled? What medications?"** **"Any recent hypoglycaemic episodes?"** **Hidden info: metformin + gliclazide. Both need to stop.**
1:30–4:00	**Medication Review**	**"I need to talk about two medications for the next 24 hours."** **"Metformin: please stop this before surgery and while you're fasting. When you're not eating normally, metformin can very rarely cause a serious condition called lactic acidosis. We'll restart it 48 hours after you're eating normally post-surgery."** **"Gliclazide: stop on the morning of surgery. When you're fasting, this can cause low blood sugar during the operation."** **Document: STOP metformin perioperatively, STOP gliclazide day of surgery.**

4:00–8:00	VRIII Explanation	**"Because you'll be fasting and having surgery, we're controlling your blood sugar with an insulin drip — called a VRIII."** **"This runs alongside a glucose drip so your blood sugar doesn't drop too low. We check your blood sugar every hour and adjust the insulin rate accordingly."** **Prescribe: VRIII with 5% glucose alongside. Write "units" never "u".** **"If blood sugar goes below 4, the nurse will pause the insulin and give you glucose. Any questions?"** *Document: metformin/gliclazide stopped, VRIII prescribed, glucose alongside, hourly monitoring plan.*

Station 15 — Self-Audit (10 points)

After your practice run, tick each item honestly. Any unticked = targeted drill needed.

#	Did you…	✓/X
1	Full diabetes history: type, duration, medications, HbA1c, recent hypos	
2	STOP metformin perioperatively (lactic acidosis risk)	
3	STOP gliclazide on day of surgery (hypoglycaemia risk)	
4	VRIII: check blood glucose before starting	
5	VRIII must run alongside glucose source (5% glucose or 0.9% NaCl + glucose)	
6	Never write insulin as "u" — write "units" in full	
7	Hourly glucose monitoring on VRIII	
8	If BG <4 on VRIII: pause infusion, give glucose, reassess	
9	Resume metformin only when eating normally post-op for 48 hours	
10	Explain plan to patient in plain language including why metformin stopped	

STATION 16

ECG / DATA INTERPRETATION (Hyperkalaemia)

Model Performance · Self-Audit Checklist · 8 Minutes

Model Performance — Top-Scoring Candidate

SAY — Bold = mark-scoring phrases · *Italic = examiner-visible actions* · **CAUTION — = instant-fail risk moment**

0:00–1:00	**Systematic ECG Read**	*ECG handed over. Read aloud immediately — do NOT stare in silence.* **"Let me read this ECG systematically. Rate — approximately 72. Rhythm — regular. P waves present. PR interval normal. QRS duration — widened, approximately 140 milliseconds. T waves — strikingly peaked in V3 to V5."** **"The combination of peaked T waves and widened QRS in a dialysis patient who has missed sessions is consistent with hyperkalaemia until proven otherwise."** **"This is a cardiac emergency."**

1:00–3:00	**Immediate Management**	**"First action: IV calcium gluconate 10% — 10mL over 2 to 3 minutes. This stabilises the heart muscle membrane. It doesn't lower the potassium, but it protects the heart. Note: calcium gluconate 10% (hyperkalaemia) ≠ calcium chloride 10% (cardiac arrest). Do not substitute."** **"Cardiac monitor, IV access, calling for senior and cardiac monitoring now."** **"Second: insulin 10 units with 50mL of 50% glucose — shifts potassium from bloodstream into cells, lowers level within 15 to 30 minutes."** **"Third: salbutamol 10mg nebulised — also shifts potassium into cells and buys more time."**

3:00–8:00	**Escalation + Definitive**	**"SBAR to renal and cardiology: Mrs Osei, 68, missed dialysis 3 days, hyperkalaemia on ECG, calcium gluconate given, insulin-dextrose in progress. Requesting emergency dialysis discussion."** **"I'm not waiting for the blood result before treating — the ECG changes tell me treatment is needed now."** **"Mrs Osei, I've found changes on your heart tracing that mean your potassium is too high. I've started treatment. The specialist team is coming."** *Document: ECG findings, calcium gluconate time, insulin-dextrose, escalation, cardiac monitoring started.*

Station 16 — Self-Audit (10 points)

After your practice run, tick each item honestly. Any unticked = targeted drill needed.

#	Did you...	✓/X
1	Read ECG systematically and ALOUD: rate, rhythm, P waves, PR, QRS, T waves	
2	Recognise: peaked T waves + wide QRS = hyperkalaemia pattern	
3	State diagnosis confidently: "Consistent with hyperkalaemia"	
4	First treatment: IV calcium gluconate 10% 10mL over 2–3 minutes (membrane stabilisation)	
5	Second: insulin 10 units + 50mL 50% dextrose (shifts K+ into cells)	

#	Did you...	✓/X
6	Third: salbutamol 10mg nebulised (temporising measure)	
7	Fourth: calcium resonium or dialysis (definitive removal)	
8	Cardiac monitoring continuously	
9	Escalate to renal/ICU for emergency dialysis discussion	
10	Do NOT give anything before calcium gluconate	

STATION 17

TELEPHONE CONSULTATION (Possible ACS)

Model Performance · Self-Audit Checklist · 8 Minutes

Model Performance — Top-Scoring Candidate

SAY — Bold = mark-scoring phrases · *Italic = examiner-visible actions* · **CAUTION — = instant-fail risk moment**

0:00–1:00	**Identify + Safety Screen**	**"Hello, this is Dr Mansour, Foundation Year 2 doctor on call. Can I take your name and date of birth? And your home address?"** **"Thank you, Mr Patel. Can you tell me what's happening? How long have you had this chest tightness? Is it there right now?"** **"Can you describe it for me? Does it go anywhere — your arm, your jaw, your back?"** **Hidden info trigger: ask directly about radiation.** **"Are you sweating? Feeling sick? Short of breath?"**
1:00–3:00	**Risk Assessment**	**"Mr Patel, I'm very concerned. Chest pain radiating to your left arm and jaw, with sweating, for 20 minutes — this is serious and needs immediate attention."** **"Any history of heart disease? Previous chest pain like this?"** **Do NOT say "it's probably nothing" or "try to rest."** **"I want to be clear with you: these symptoms could indicate a heart attack. This needs to be assessed in hospital immediately."**

3:00–8:00	999 + Stay on Line	**"I need you to call 999 for an ambulance right now. Do not drive yourself and do not let anyone drive you."** Critical fail trigger: advising patient to drive or take a taxi. **"Can you do that for me now? I can stay on the line with you until you've called."** **"Can you also unlock your front door so the paramedics can get in quickly? And if you have aspirin in the house and you're not allergic, chew one adult aspirin while you wait."** **"I'm documenting this call and alerting the ED. Please call 999 now."** *Document: time of call, symptoms, advice (999, do not drive), aspirin advised, ED alerted.*

Station 17 — Self-Audit (10 points)

After your practice run, tick each item honestly. Any unticked = targeted drill needed.

#	Did you...	✓/X
1	Identify yourself fully: name, role, grade	
2	Confirm patient identity: full name, DOB, home address	
3	Establish urgency: when did symptoms start, current severity	
4	Safety screen: chest pain + sweating + radiation = high risk	
5	Do NOT tell patient to drive to hospital — critical fail trigger	
6	Do NOT tell patient to wait for GP tomorrow	
7	Advise: call 999 immediately for ambulance	
8	Stay on phone until patient confirms ambulance called	
9	Advise unlock front door for paramedics	
10	Document: time of call, symptoms, advice given, 999 confirmed	

STATION 18

ANGRY RELATIVE (Duty of Candour)

Model Performance · Self-Audit Checklist · 8 Minutes

Model Performance — Top-Scoring Candidate

SAY — Bold = mark-scoring phrases · *Italic = examiner-visible actions* · **CAUTION — = instant-fail risk moment**

0:00–1:00	**Private Room + Listen**	*Do NOT start in corridor. "Mrs Clarke, I want to speak with you properly. Can we find a quiet room?"* **"Hello Mrs Clarke, I'm Dr Mansour, one of the doctors looking after your father. Thank you for coming to speak with me."** **"I understand you have serious concerns. I want to hear everything. Please take your time."** *Sit down. Eye contact. No phone. Let her speak without interrupting.*
1:00–3:00	**Acknowledge + Genuine Apology**	**"Mrs Clarke, I want to start by saying: I'm sorry. I'm sorry that your father waited six hours and that a pressure sore has developed. Regardless of the circumstances, that was not the experience he deserved."** **NEVER say: "I'm sorry you feel that way." Conditional apology = instant fail.** **"A six-hour wait and a pressure sore are things we take seriously. I can hear how worried you are about your father."**
3:00–5:30	**Explain + Duty of Candour**	**"I want to be as honest as I can. A pressure sore can develop when a patient is in one position for too long without repositioning. I'm not offering you a reason that sounds like an excuse."** **"The pressure sore will be reviewed by our tissue viability nurse today. I'm documenting this conversation and making sure it goes to the right people for review."** **"Under the Duty of Candour we are required to acknowledge when things have gone wrong and tell you what we are doing about it. I want to honour that."** **Do NOT say "this will never happen again" — you cannot guarantee this.**
5:30–8:00	**Next Steps + PALS**	**"Your father is having his surgery tomorrow morning. He is stable. The surgical team are aware of his situation."** **"If you'd like a formal investigation, I can refer you to PALS — the Patient Advice and Liaison Service. They can take your complaint further independently."** **"Is there anything else I can do right now to help you?"** *Document: relative spoken to, concerns heard, genuine apology given, Duty of Candour fulfilled, action plan, PALS offered.*

Station 18 — Self-Audit (10 points)

After your practice run, tick each item honestly. Any unticked = targeted drill needed.

#	Did you...	✓/X
1	Find a private room BEFORE beginning any conversation	
2	Introduce name, role, grade clearly	
3	Let relative speak first — do not interrupt or defend	
4	Acknowledge the complaint genuinely before any explanation	

#	Did you...	✓/X
5	Genuine apology: "I am sorry this happened" NOT "I'm sorry you feel that way"	
6	Duty of Candour: acknowledge incident, apologise, explain, commit to improvement	
7	Do NOT be defensive or blame other team members	
8	Do NOT make promises you cannot keep	
9	Explain what happens next: investigation, feedback loop	
10	Offer PALS if formal resolution wanted	

TOP 5 EXAMINER Q&A · BLOOD TESTS & CLINICAL REASONING	
Q1. How do you read a panel without drowning?	Scan systematically, flag the dangerous values first (potassium, glucose, pH-related), then build one story that explains the pattern.
Q2. Hyponatraemia: the first two questions?	How fast and how symptomatic: acute symptomatic needs senior help and careful hypertonic-saline territory: chronic is corrected slowly.
Q3. The potassium values that change your next 10 minutes?	6.0–6.5 with changes, or 6.5 and above regardless: ECG, calcium gluconate, insulin-dextrose: now.
Q4. A raised troponin always means MI?	No: interpret with the clinical picture and the dynamic change: sepsis, PE, renal failure and tachyarrhythmias all raise it.
Q5. How do you present multi-domain results?	One synthesis sentence: "the anaemia, renal impairment and raised calcium together suggest myeloma: I would request…": integration is the skill.
CURVEBALL	Two abnormalities point in opposite directions. Say it explicitly: name the conflict, the unifying possibilities, and the test that discriminates: examiners are marking exactly this moment.

Appendix 3E

SAFEGUARDING & LEGAL FRAMEWORKS — PLAB 2 RAPID REFERENCE

CORE · HIGH INSTANT FAIL RISK · VULNERABLE PATIENTS · RECOGNITION · ESCALATION

Safeguarding stations test whether you can:
▸ Recognise risk · ▸ Protect the patient immediately · ▸ Speak safely and professionally
▸ Maintain confidentiality appropriately · ▸ Escalate without delay · ▸ Understand capacity and consent

Most candidates fail because they:
Promise confidentiality · Ignore safeguarding clues · Speak in front of controlling relatives
Forget capacity assessment · Do not escalate · Confuse MCA vs MHA · Miss mandatory reporting duties

Golden Rule of Safeguarding

Step	Action
1	Ensure immediate safety
2	Treat urgent medical problems first
3	Speak to the patient ALONE
4	Use open, non-judgemental questions
5	Document VERBATIM using quotation marks
6	Never promise confidentiality
7	Escalate immediately to safeguarding lead
8	Follow local safeguarding policy

THINK — Universal Safeguarding Script:
"I am concerned this patient may be at risk. I will ensure immediate safety, speak to them alone in a safe environment, document exactly what they tell me using their own words, and escalate to the safeguarding lead immediately. I cannot promise complete confidentiality if someone is at risk of harm."
Mantra: When in doubt, escalate. It is safer to raise a safeguarding concern than to miss one.

Non-Negotiable Safeguarding Rules

INSTANT FAIL NEVER	✓ ALWAYS
Promise confidentiality	Explain safeguarding limits clearly
Question aggressively	Use calm, open questions
Ignore controlling relatives	Speak to patient alone
Document opinions as facts	Record objective findings
Delay escalation	Escalate early
Assume lack of capacity	Presume capacity first
Use family as interpreter	Use professional interpreter
Ignore concern because evidence incomplete	Raise concern if worried

Mental Capacity Act 2005 (MCA)

Applies to: Adults aged 16+ · Decision-specific capacity assessment

Principle	OSCE Script
1. Presume capacity	"I start from the assumption this patient has capacity."
2. Support decision-making	"I will support communication using simple language, interpreters, advocates, or written information."
3. Unwise ≠ incapacity	"A decision that seems unwise does not automatically mean the patient lacks capacity."
4. Best interests	"If capacity is lacking, I will act in the patient's best interests."
5. Least restrictive	"I will choose the least restrictive safe option."

Capacity Assessment — 2-Stage Test:

Stage 1 — Diagnostic: Is there impairment or disturbance of mind/brain? (delirium, dementia, psychosis, intoxication, learning disability, head injury)
Stage 2 — Functional: Can they Understand · Retain · Weigh · Communicate?
SAY — Script: "I need to assess whether there is an impairment of mind or brain, and whether this prevents the patient from understanding, retaining, weighing, or communicating this specific decision."

Common MCA Fails:
Assuming confused = no capacity · Not reassessing (capacity fluctuates) · Ignoring communication barriers
Forgetting best interests · Using restraint unnecessarily

Deprivation of Liberty Safeguards (DoLS)

Applies to: Adults 18+ · Lacking capacity · Hospital or care home

Think DoLS if: Continuous supervision · Not free to leave · Restrictions required for safety

SAY — Script: "This patient lacks capacity, is under continuous supervision, and is not free to leave. I would check whether a DoLS authorisation is in place and escalate appropriately."

Outside hospital/care home: Court of Protection / Liberty Protection Safeguards pathway. No deep legal detail required in PLAB 2.

Mental Health Act 1983 (MHA)

MCA = Decision-making capacity · MHA = Detention/treatment for mental disorder when risk is significant

Section	Purpose	Duration	Script
Section 2	Assessment	Up to 28 days	"Section 2 is used for assessment."
Section 3	Treatment	6 months renewable	"Section 3 is used for ongoing treatment."
Section 4	Emergency assessment	Up to 72h	"Section 4 for urgent situations where delay is unsafe."
Section 5(2)	Doctor holding power	72h	"Doctor can stop inpatient leaving temporarily."
Section 5(4)	Nurse holding power	6h	"Nurse may temporarily prevent at-risk inpatient leaving."
Section 136	Police power	Variable	"Police may remove from public place to place of safety."

MHA High-Fail Confusions:

Using MHA for physical illness only · Confusing MCA (capacity) with MHA (detention)

Forgetting least restrictive approach · Detaining voluntary patients casually

Children & Young People — Gillick & Fraser

Term	Applies To
Gillick Competence	ANY medical decision for child <16 — assess sufficient understanding and maturity
Fraser Guidelines	Contraception / sexual health specifically — all 5 criteria must be met

SAY — Gillick Script: "I need to assess whether this child has sufficient understanding and maturity to make this decision."

Fraser — Contraception (<16) requires all 5: Child understands advice · Cannot be persuaded to involve parents · Likely to continue sexual activity · Health may suffer otherwise · Treatment in best interests

Age	General Rule
0–11	Usually parental involvement
11–15	Assess Gillick competency
16+	Presumed competent

> Safeguarding overrides confidentiality. You MUST escalate if:
> Child at risk · Vulnerable adult at risk · Serious harm risk · FGM concerns · Significant domestic abuse · Modern slavery · Radicalisation

High-Yield Safeguarding Topics

Topic	RED FLAGS	Script
FGM	Disclosure · Exam findings · Family history · Planned travel abroad	"Girl <18 and FGM identified → mandatory reporting immediately."
Domestic Abuse	Controlling partner · Inconsistent story · Fearful behaviour · Delayed presentation	"Are you safe? Has anyone hurt, threatened, or controlled you?"
Modern Slavery	No documents · Fearful · Someone answering for patient · Restricted movement	"I will escalate to safeguarding and consider NRM referral."
PREVENT	Extremist influence · Isolation · Sudden behavioural change · Vulnerability	"I will discuss with safeguarding and Prevent leads → consider Channel referral."
Elder Abuse	Pressure ulcers · Financial concerns · Carer intimidation · Medication neglect	"I will ensure safety, speak to patient alone, document objectively, and escalate."

Safeguarding RED FLAGS by Group

Adults	Children	Elderly
Delayed presentation	Bruises in non-mobile child	Pressure ulcers
Inconsistent story	Recurrent injuries	Poor hygiene
Fearful behaviour	Withdrawal	Malnutrition
Controlling partner	Developmental concerns	Financial exploitation
Neglect signs	Unsafe home	Carer burnout

Documentation Rules

✓ Document	✗ Never Document
Exact words in quotation marks	Personal opinions
Objective injuries	Assumptions
Body maps if required	Accusatory language
Time/date · Who was present	Unverified hearsay
Escalation actions taken	

SAY — Documentation Script: "I will document the history, examination findings, exact patient statements, safeguarding concerns, capacity assessment, escalation, and safety plan clearly and objectively."

✓ 11 Safeguarding Behaviours That Score Marks

1 Presume capacity first · 2 Speak to vulnerable patients alone · 3 Use professional interpreters
4 Explain confidentiality limits · 5 Document verbatim · 6 Escalate early
7 Recognise domestic abuse red flags · 8 Recognise modern slavery indicators
9 Know FGM mandatory escalation · 10 Understand Gillick vs Fraser · 11 Use best-interests framework

Final Exam Mantras

Safeguarding: Safety first → Speak alone → Document verbatim → Escalate
Capacity: Understand → Retain → Weigh → Communicate
MCA: Presume capacity first
MHA: Risk + mental disorder + legal detention

Gold Closing Statement:
"I have assessed the patient's immediate safety, capacity, and safeguarding risk. I will document concerns clearly, escalate appropriately to the safeguarding team, and ensure ongoing support and follow-up. If capacity is lacking, I will act in the patient's best interests using the least restrictive safe approach."

Before ending ANY safeguarding station, verify:
✓ Immediate safety · ✓ Capacity assessment · ✓ Speaking to patient alone
✓ Documentation · ✓ Escalation · ✓ Follow-up

Never promise confidentiality in safeguarding	Speak alone always with vulnerable patients	Document verbatim quotation marks	Escalate early when in doubt, escalate	Presume capacity MCA Principle 1
4 functions understand retain weigh communicate	Gillick any medical decision <16	Fraser contraception only <16	FGM <18 mandatory reporting	MCA vs MHA capacity vs detention

Appendix 3F

NHS VOCABULARY & COMMUNICATION STYLE FOR IMGs

UK Clinical Language Orientation for PLAB 2 & UKMLA CPSA

CORE · HIGH INSTANT FAIL RISK · COMMUNICATION MARKS · NHS CULTURE · IMG SURVIVAL GUIDE

Why This Appendix 3Fxists:
Many IMGs know the medicine well but lose marks because their communication sounds:
Too formal · Too direct · Too robotic · Too medical · Too authoritarian · Not patient-centred · Missing NHS vocabulary

🔴 Core NHS Communication Principle: Complex medical vocabulary is NOT rewarded. Clear explanation IS rewarded.

Golden Formula: Simple words → Clear explanation → Check understanding

High-Fail IMG Language Errors

Less Natural (Avoid)	✓ Better NHS Style
"What is your complaint?"	"What brings you in today?"
"Kindly sit."	"Please have a seat."
"Cooperate with treatment."	"Work with us on the treatment plan."
"You failed treatment."	"The treatment has not helped enough yet."
"You are non-compliant."	"You've had difficulty following the treatment."
"Calm down."	"I can see this is distressing."
"You must lose weight."	"Losing weight could really help your symptoms."
"You need admission."	"I think the safest option would be admission."
"There is nothing wrong."	"The tests are reassuring."
"Negative result."	"The test did not show anything concerning."
"Obese patient."	"Patient with obesity."
"Diabetic patient."	"Patient with diabetes."
"Why didn't you come earlier?"	"What made you decide to come in today?"

Words That Can Lose Marks

Avoid	✓ Use Instead
"Complaint"	"Concern" / "symptom"

Avoid	✓ Use Instead
"Failed"	"Has not improved"
"Refused"	"Decided not to"
"Poor historian"	"History limited"
"Drug addict"	"Person with substance misuse"
"Alcoholic"	"Alcohol dependence"
"Crazy"	"Mental health difficulties"
"Terminal" (abruptly)	"Serious / life-limiting illness"

NHS Softening Language — Very High Yield

Direct (Avoid)	NHS Style (✓)
"You need surgery."	"I think surgery may be the best option."
"Stop smoking."	"I'd strongly recommend stopping smoking."
"You cannot drive."	"You should avoid driving until we confirm it is safe."
"You are depressed."	"You may be experiencing symptoms of depression."
"This is cancer."	"The results are concerning for cancer."
"You are wrong."	"I understand why you think that."

THINK — High-Yield NHS Phrases

Purpose	Phrase
Opening	"What brings you in today?" · "Tell me what's been happening." · "Take your time."
Empathy	"I can see this has been difficult." · "That sounds very worrying." · "I'm sorry you've been going through this."
Explaining	"Let me explain this in simple terms." · "I'll explain this step by step."
Checking understanding	"Does that make sense so far?" · "Would you like me to go over that again?"
Shared decision-making	"We'll decide this together." · "How do you feel about that plan?"
Escalation & Safety	"I'll discuss this with my senior." · "I do not want to delay treatment."

NHS Healthcare Roles

Role	Meaning
GP	General practitioner (community doctor)
Consultant	Most senior specialist doctor
Registrar	Senior specialty trainee
Core Trainee (CT)	Early specialty training doctor
FY1/FY2	Foundation doctor
ANP	Advanced Nurse Practitioner
CNS	Clinical Nurse Specialist
HCA	Healthcare Assistant
Ward clerk	Administrative ward staff
Bed manager	Coordinates hospital beds

NHS System Navigation · Ward Language · Clinical Areas

Term	Meaning	Example
A&E	Emergency department	"I'll refer you to A&E."
AMU	Acute Medical Unit	"Admitted to AMU."
Bleep	Pager call	"I'll bleep the registrar."
On-call	Emergency duty shift	"The on-call team will review you."
Board round	Daily patient review meeting	"Your case is on today's board round."
Handover	Transfer of clinical responsibility	"I'll hand this over to the night team."
TTO	To Take Out (discharge prescription)	CRITICAL — every discharge station
NEWS2	National Early Warning Score (0–20; ≥5 = urgent)	Sepsis, deterioration
DNACPR	Do Not Attempt CPR	Resuscitation decision
Safety-netting	Advice if symptoms worsen	"I've safety-netted the patient."

Critical Clinical Abbreviations — Must Know

INSTANT FAIL Never say these to patients without explanation. Use plain English when speaking.

Abbreviation	Meaning	Notes
TTO	To Take Out (discharge prescription)	CRITICAL — every discharge station
DNACPR	Do Not Attempt CPR	Resuscitation decision
ReSPECT	Recommended Summary Plan for Emergency Care and Treatment	Newer DNACPR framework
NEWS2	National Early Warning Score (0–20; ≥5 = urgent review)	Sepsis, deterioration
AKI	Acute kidney injury	Urology, nephrology, sepsis
CSU	Catheter specimen of urine	Urology, infection
LRTI/URTI	Lower/Upper respiratory tract infection	Respiratory
CVA/TIA	Cerebrovascular accident / Transient ischaemic attack	Neurology
DVT/PE	Deep vein thrombosis / Pulmonary embolism	Haematology, respiratory
D/W	Discussed with	Handover documentation
F/U	Follow-up	Outpatient planning
Hx / Rx	History / Treatment/prescription	Notes shorthand

SAY — Patient Colloquial Language — Clinical Meaning

Patient Phrase	Clinical Meaning
"My chest feels tight / heavy."	Chest pain/pressure — possible cardiac
"My heart was racing."	Palpitations
"I nearly blacked out."	Near syncope
"My legs are puffy."	Leg oedema
"Food gets stuck."	Dysphagia
"I'm passing water a lot."	Urinary frequency
"I'm peeing blood."	Haematuria
"It burns when I pee."	Dysuria
"I can't pee at all."	Urinary retention
"I'm wheezy."	Wheeze / airway narrowing

Patient Phrase	Clinical Meaning
"I'm bunged up."	Constipation / nasal blockage
"I'm bringing up blood."	Haemoptysis
"I'm pooing blood."	PR bleeding / melaena

Patient-Friendly Medical Language

Medical Term	Patient-Friendly Language
Dyspnoea	Shortness of breath
Syncope	Fainting
Haematemesis	Vomiting blood
Oedema	Swelling
Hypertension	High blood pressure
Fracture	Broken bone
Benign/Malignant	Non-cancerous / Cancerous
Myocardial infarction	Heart attack

SAY — Always say: "In simple terms, what this means is…"

Generic vs Brand Medication Names

Generic	Brand	Notes
Paracetamol	Panadol	Common analgesic
Salbutamol	Ventolin	Asthma inhaler / nebuliser
Omeprazole	Losec	PPI for acid reflux
Metformin	Glucophage	Diabetes
Atorvastatin	Lipitor	Cholesterol
Adrenaline	EpiPen (auto-injector)	Anaphylaxis — emergency
Lorazepam	(UK uses generic)	Status epilepticus
Midazolam	Buccolam (buccal)	Seizures — no IV access
Insulin aspart	Novorapid	Rapid-acting insulin

Generic	Brand	Notes
Insulin glargine	Lantus	Long-acting insulin

NHS Documentation Language

Term	Meaning
"Safety-netted"	Advice given if symptoms worsen
"Clinically stable"	No immediate deterioration
"For senior review"	Needs escalation
"Medically fit for discharge"	Safe to leave hospital
"Mobilising independently"	Walking safely alone
"Tolerating oral intake"	Eating/drinking adequately
"TTOs written"	Discharge prescriptions completed

Core Communication Rules for PLAB 2

✓ ALWAYS	INSTANT FAIL NEVER
Use plain English	Overuse jargon
Speak naturally	Sound robotic
Explain step by step	Speak aggressively or judgementally
Check understanding	Lecture patients
Use empathy	Use unexplained abbreviations
Involve patients	Miss TTO/DNACPR/NEWS2 in context
Know key clinical terms for notes/handover	Sound overly formal

Final Exam Mantras

Communication Formula: Simple → Clear → Kind → Check understanding
NHS Style: Collaborative, not authoritarian
Clinical Vocabulary Rule: Know the term for notes (TTO, DNACPR, NEWS2, CSU). Explain in plain English to patients.
PLAB 2 Rule: Natural communication scores more highly than complex vocabulary.

Gold Closing Statement:

"I will explain things clearly using simple language, check the patient's understanding, involve them in decisions, and communicate in a calm, respectful, patient-centred way. I will use appropriate clinical terminology when speaking with colleagues and document clearly using standard NHS abbreviations."

Plain English first not medical jargon	Know TTO every discharge station	Know NEWS2 ≥5 = urgent review	Know DNACPR resuscitation decision	Softening language collaborative not authoritarian
Check understanding chunk and check always	Empathy phrases I can see this is difficult	Shared decisions how do you feel about that?	Colloquial terms know what patients mean	Safe doctors pass clear communication is key

Appendix 3G

ADAPTING TO UK CLINICAL CULTURE

Communication Norms & Professional Expectations for PLAB 2 / UKMLA CPSA

PATIENT-CENTRED · EMPATHY & ICE · ESCALATION · CONSENT & CAPACITY · SAFEGUARDING · EXAMINER MINDSET

Purpose: Equip IMGs with a clear understanding of how UK clinical culture works in real NHS practice and within OSCE-style assessments.

Focus Areas: Patient-centred communication · Shared decision-making · Consent & capacity · Safeguarding · Escalation & hierarchy · Documentation culture · Structured communication · Examiner mindset · IMG-specific pitfalls

1 Patient-Centred Communication (ICE)

UK consultations prioritise the patient's perspective. Non-negotiable and consistently assessed.

ICE Questions:

Ideas: "What do you think might be causing this?"

Concerns: "Is there anything in particular you're worried about?"

Expectations: "What were you hoping we could do today?"

Opening: "Hello, I'm one of the doctors. What brings you in today?"

Expected Behaviours:

✓ Warm introduction · ✓ Open questions before narrowing · ✓ Active listening without interruption

✓ Acknowledge emotions · ✓ Clear explanations · ✓ Involve the patient in decisions

2 Shared Decision-Making

Patients are partners, not passive recipients.

✓ Explain all reasonable options · ✓ Discuss risks & benefits · ✓ Explore patient preferences · ✓ Agree collaboratively on a plan

SAY — Example: "We can decide together what would work best for you."

3 Professional Escalation & Hierarchy

Escalation = safe clinical judgement, not weakness.

When to Escalate: Diagnostic uncertainty · Abnormal observations · Concerns about capacity or safety · Situations beyond your competence

SAY — Phrases: "I would discuss this with my senior." · "I would escalate this to the consultant." · "I would request specialist review."

4 Capacity & Consent

Capacity = Ability to: Understand · Retain · Weigh · Communicate a choice
If lacking capacity → best interests decision + senior involvement.
Consent must be: informed, voluntary, and capacity-dependent.
SAY — Example: "It's your choice whether to proceed. I'll explain the options first."

5 Safeguarding Awareness

Recognise and escalate safeguarding concerns promptly.
Key Areas: Child protection · Domestic abuse · Neglect of vulnerable adults · Patients unable to protect themselves
SAY — Example: "I would escalate this concern to the safeguarding team."
CAUTION — Failing to recognise safeguarding triggers = high OSCE fail risk.

6 Documentation Culture

NHS documentation must be clear, factual, and contemporaneous.
Include: History & examination · Discussion with patient · Capacity/consent assessment · Management plan & follow-up
SAY — Example: "I would document the discussion, findings, and plan clearly in the notes."

7 Structured Communication

Technique	**Example**
Signpost	"I'm going to ask a few questions about your symptoms."
Chunk	Give information in digestible sections — pause between each
Check understanding	"Does that make sense?"
Verbalise reasoning	"I would first check your observations and discuss any concerns with my senior."

Structured talk = structured thinking = higher scores.

8 Empathy & Emotional Validation

Explicitly acknowledge patient emotions. Empathy is a scored domain.
"That sounds very difficult." · "I can see this is worrying for you." · "Thank you for sharing that."
"Would you feel more comfortable with a chaperone or another clinician present?"

9 Safety-First Clinical Decision-Making

NHS prioritises safety over diagnostic certainty.

Safety-First Behaviours: Investigate appropriately · Seek senior advice early · Arrange follow-up · Provide clear safety-netting

SAY — Safety-net phrase: "If symptoms worsen, new symptoms appear, or you feel concerned, please seek medical help urgently."

Examiner Mindset

Core Question: "Would I trust this doctor to practise safely in the NHS?"

Examiners REWARD ✓	Examiners PENALISE ✗
Clear communication	Ignoring concerns
Shared decision-making	Rushed or unclear explanations
Empathy	Unilateral decisions
Appropriate escalation	Failure to escalate uncertainty
Verbalised reasoning	Dismissiveness or paternalism

Clinical behaviour is assessed as much as medical knowledge.

DISTINCTION — Rewarded vs Penalised — At a Glance

✓ Rewarded	✗ Penalised
Introduce yourself warmly	No greeting, abrupt start
Open questions first	Closed questions only
Acknowledge patient concerns	Dismiss or minimise concerns
Explain in plain English	Use jargon
Involve patient in decisions	Make unilateral decisions
Escalate when unsure	Avoid escalation
Provide clear safety-net	No safety-netting
Verbalise reasoning	Stay silent during tasks
Acknowledge emotions	Ignore patient distress

Common IMG Mistakes — Quick Corrections

Less Natural (Avoid)	More Natural (UK)
"What is your complaint?"	"What brings you in today?"
"Kindly sit down."	"Please have a seat."
"Kindly cooperate."	"Could you work with me?"
"I will check you."	"I'll examine you."
"Tell me your problem."	"Tell me what's been happening."
"Don't worry."	"I understand this is worrying."
"You must do this."	"I would recommend this."

Key Messages — High-Yield Summary

Core Cultural Rule: ✓ Empathy · ✓ Clarity · ✓ Collaboration · ✓ Patient Safety
ICE: Ask early, revisit often
Escalate: "I would discuss this with my senior."
Empathy: "That sounds very difficult."
Safety-net: "If symptoms worsen, please seek medical help urgently."
🔴 Final Rule: Behave like a safe NHS doctor — that is what passes the exam.

Final Takeaway:
"Every station is an opportunity to demonstrate safe, empathetic, collaborative NHS behaviour. The exam is not testing whether you sound British — it is testing whether you behave like a safe NHS doctor."
ICE + Escalation + Empathy + Safety-net = your exam anchors

ICE always ask early, revisit often	Open questions first what brings you in?	Shared decisions we decide together	Escalate early not a weakness	Acknowledge emotions empathy is scored
Safety-net every station if symptoms worsen...	Verbalise reasoning structured talk = marks	Plain English never jargon to patients	Document clearly factual, contemporaneous	Safe NHS doctor that is what passes

Appendix 3H · HOW CANDIDATES ACTUALLY FAIL · MARK SHEET · PLAB 2 vs UKMLA

10 Behavioural Fail Vignettes · Examiner Mark Sheet Walkthrough · PLAB 2 vs UKMLA Comparison

AMaC (A. Mansour and Colleagues) · PLAB 2 Master Series

How Candidates Actually Fail — 10 Real Vignettes

These vignettes are based on examiner feedback and PLAB 2 circuit recall reports. All names and details are anonymised composites.

Read them once. The patterns are more important than the details. Every single one of these fails was preventable.

Vignette 1: The Knowledge Trap

Scenario: Acute chest pain station. Patient has SpO_2 of 84%, diaphoretic, looks unwell.

What happened: Candidate took a detailed smoking history, occupational history, and family history for 4 minutes. Never gave oxygen. Never escalated. Finished the history as time ended.

Why it failed: ABCDE was never initiated. Examiner marked: "No immediate management of unwell patient." Patient safety domain: fail.

✓ Lesson: **When a patient looks unwell: STOP the history. ABCDE first. Oxygen. Call for help. History can wait.**

Vignette 2: The Conditional Apology

Scenario: Complaint station. Patient unhappy about a medication error on the ward.

What happened: Candidate said: "I'm sorry you feel that way." Then explained the error was "unlikely to cause harm." Did not acknowledge duty of candour.

Why it failed: "Sorry you feel that way" is not an apology. It is a conditional statement that dismisses the patient's experience. Examiner marked: "No genuine apology. No duty of candour."

✓ Lesson: **Duty of candour requires: acknowledge the incident · give a genuine apology · explain what happened · say what will be done. "I am sorry this happened" not "I am sorry you feel that way."**

Vignette 3: The Promised Secret

Scenario: 14-year-old discloses father hitting her during a consultation for a sports injury.

What happened: Candidate said: "I promise this will stay between us." Took history. Did not mention safeguarding. Closed the station normally.

Why it failed: Promising confidentiality to a child in a safeguarding situation is an instant fail. The examiner's marking note: "Promised secrecy to a vulnerable child. No safeguarding escalation."

✓ Lesson: **Never promise secrecy in any situation. In safeguarding: acknowledge the disclosure · say you have a duty to share this · escalate to safeguarding team · do NOT promise it will stay private.**

Vignette 4: The Diagnosis Without The Empathy

Scenario: Breaking bad news — explaining a new cancer diagnosis.

What happened: Candidate delivered the diagnosis clearly and accurately. Used the word "cancer". Gave a management plan. Offered follow-up. Did not pause after delivering the news. Did not acknowledge the patient's emotional response. Patient was visibly crying.

Why it failed: Clinical content was correct. Communication domain failed. "Candidate continued speaking while patient cried. No acknowledgement of distress. No empathy phrases used."

✓ **Lesson: When a patient cries: STOP speaking. Pause. Acknowledge. "This is clearly very difficult news. Take all the time you need." Clinical content means nothing if you deliver it over someone's grief.**

Vignette 5: The Ignored Refusal

Scenario: Patient refusing blood transfusion on religious grounds. Haemoglobin 62 g/L.

What happened: Candidate explained the risks clearly. Patient still refused. Candidate said: "I strongly advise you to accept the transfusion" three times. Called it "reckless." Then said they would transfuse anyway.

Why it failed: Mental Capacity Act violation. Patient had capacity. Informed refusal must be respected regardless of clinical risk. Instant fail on the capacity and consent domain.

✓ **Lesson: Capacity + informed refusal = patient's right regardless of clinical risk. Your role: ensure they understand the consequences · document the decision · respect it · arrange alternatives where possible.**

Vignette 6: The Daily Methotrexate

Scenario: Prescribing station. Patient with rheumatoid arthritis. Drug chart shows methotrexate 10mg daily.

What happened: Candidate prescribed it without questioning the frequency. Counselled the patient on taking it "every day with food."

Why it failed: Methotrexate prescribed daily is a prescribing safety fail. Frequency error not spotted. Counselling reinforced the error. Examiner note: "Failed to identify and correct a potentially fatal prescribing error."

✓ **Lesson: Any time you see methotrexate on a drug chart: confirm ONCE WEEKLY before prescribing or counselling. If the chart says daily, say "I would not prescribe this as written — methotrexate must be ONCE WEEKLY."**

Vignette 7: The Silent Freeze

Scenario: Data interpretation station. ABG results handed to candidate.

What happened: Candidate looked at the results for 35 seconds in silence. Examiner prompted: "What do you think?" Candidate said: "I'm not sure." More silence.

Why it failed: Silence is not a safe behaviour in PLAB 2. Examiner cannot mark reasoning they cannot hear. Examiner note: "No verbalisation of findings. No systematic approach demonstrated."

✓ **Lesson: When given data: start talking immediately. "Let me look at this systematically." Then: pH · $PaCO_2$ · HCO_3 · oxygenation. Even if uncertain, a structured attempt scores higher than silence.**

Vignette 8: The Overcrowded History

Scenario: History of presenting complaint station. Patient with abdominal pain.

What happened: Candidate asked 47 questions in 8 minutes. SOCRATES completed. Systems review completed. All red flags asked. Patient's ideas, concerns, and expectations never asked. Patient said their main concern was cancer. Candidate did not hear this.

Why it failed: Communication and ICE domain failed. "Candidate focused entirely on clinical content. Patient's main concern was never addressed. No empathy demonstrated."

✓ **Lesson: ICE is not optional and it is not at the end. Ask early: "What do you think might be causing this? What worries you most?" A patient who volunteers the word "cancer" is giving you the station on a plate.**

Vignette 9: The DVLA Breach

Scenario: Ethics station. Patient with newly diagnosed epilepsy insists they will keep driving.

What happened: Candidate explained the DVLA rules. Patient refused to stop driving. Candidate said: "In that case I'll have to call the police."

Why it failed: The correct route is DVLA notification, not the police. The candidate confused the breach of confidentiality framework. Examiner note: "Incorrect breach pathway. No documentation discussed."

✓ **Lesson: DVLA breach pathway: advise patient to inform DVLA · if they refuse, you may inform DVLA directly · document your decision · inform the patient you are doing so. Never threaten police.**

Vignette 10: The Near Miss They Passed

Scenario: Same acute chest pain station as Vignette 1. Different candidate.

What happened: Candidate looked at the patient, said: "You look unwell. I'm going to stop our conversation for a moment. I need to check your vital signs and ensure you're safe first." Applied ABCDE. Called for help. Gave oxygen. Then returned to history. Scored in the top 20% of the circuit.

Why it failed: Did not know the diagnosis. Did not complete the history. Passed because they demonstrated the most important competency in PLAB 2: prioritising patient safety over clinical completeness.

✓ **Lesson: Safety before completeness. Always. Every time. Without exception.**

The Pattern Across All 10 Vignettes:

Not one candidate failed because they lacked clinical knowledge. Every single fail was a behaviour: ignored safety · missed empathy · wrong framework · silence · rushed past ICE · promised what they could not promise.

PLAB 2 is a behaviour test with clinical content in it. Not a clinical test with some behaviour in it.

Examiner Mark Sheet Walkthrough — How Marks Are Actually Awarded

Most candidates have never seen a PLAB 2 mark sheet. Understanding how marks are allocated changes how you prepare.

The GMC uses a structured mark sheet with domains. Each domain is scored independently. You can fail one domain and still pass the station if other domains compensate — except safety, which is an instant fail regardless.

Generic OSCE Mark Sheet Structure — All Station Types

Domain	Marks (typical)	What Triggers a Tick
Introduction + consent	1–2	Name · role · purpose of consultation · permission to proceed
ICE — Ideas, Concerns, Expectations	2–4	All three components asked · patient's response acknowledged · revisited mid-consultation
History / Clinical assessment	4–6	Systematic approach · relevant questions asked · red flags explored
Communication skills	3–5	Empathy language · signposting · chunk + check · clear language · no jargon
Clinical management	3–5	Appropriate diagnosis discussed · management plan reasonable · investigations logical
Shared decision-making	1–2	Options offered · patient preference explored · not imposed
Safety-netting	1–2	Specific red flags given · when to return stated · personalised to this patient
Escalation / Documentation	1–2	Senior involvement stated · documentation mentioned · follow-up arranged
PATIENT SAFETY (Global)	AUTO FAIL	Any safety breach = station fail regardless of other marks

History Station:
Mark allocation: ICE (4 marks) + Clinical Assessment (6 marks) = 10/20 minimum from just these two
✓ **Key insight:** Candidates who ask all of SOCRATES but skip ICE lose 4 marks instantly. ICE alone is worth more than the entire systems review.

Examination Station:
Mark allocation: Systematic technique (5) + Correct findings verbalised (5) + Communication (4) + Safety (global)
✓ **Key insight:** Silence kills examination stations. Examiners cannot mark what they cannot hear. Verbalise every single step and every finding, even normal ones.

Prescribing Station:
Mark allocation: Allergy check (2) + Correct drug/dose/frequency (4) + Counselling + teach-back (4) + Monitoring (2) + Safety (global)
✓ **Key insight:** Allergy check = 2 free marks. Takes 5 seconds. Never skip it. MTX/insulin errors = safety fail regardless of other marks.

Explanation Station:
Mark allocation: Chunking + checking understanding (3) + ICE during explanation (3) + Written info offered (1) + Safety-net (2)

✓ **Key insight:** Most candidates explain correctly but forget to CHECK understanding. "What have you understood so far?" = 3 marks for one question.

Challenging Communication:
Mark allocation: Empathy language (4) + Not arguing/bridging (3) + ICE deep dive (3) + Collaborative plan (3)

✓ **Key insight:** Do not argue. Do not lecture. Do not repeat yourself louder. Bridge: "I understand. Can I share some information?" = examiner tick.

Data Interpretation:
Mark allocation: Systematic approach verbalised (4) + Correct interpretation (4) + Management plan (4) + Escalation (2)

✓ **Key insight:** Say the mnemonic aloud: "pH first... $PaCO_2$ next..." Examiners mark the process, not just the answer.

The Safety Domain is Different From All Others:
Every other domain: marks accumulate. Safety: binary. One breach = station fail regardless of total marks.
Safety breaches include: no escalation for unwell patient · prescribing despite allergy · sending suicidal patient home without safety plan · overriding informed refusal · ignoring safeguarding disclosure.

PLAB 2 vs UKMLA CPSA — What's the Difference?

This series is fully aligned with both PLAB 2 and the UKMLA Clinical and Professional Skills Assessment (CPSA). The differences below are minor — the core system is identical.

Domain	PLAB 2	UKMLA CPSA
Format	18 stations · 8 minutes each	18 stations · 8 minutes each
Station types	History · Examination · Procedure · Explanation · Prescribing · Data · Communication	Same types · Same structure
Core emphasis	Safety · ICE · Escalation · Professionalism	Same · Plus explicit EDI (Equality, Diversity, Inclusion) scoring
Paediatrics	Adult-focused · Paeds stations ~10–15%	Paeds stations slightly more frequent (~20%)
Prescribing	Drug chart · dose calculations · safety	Same · Antibiotic stewardship 48–72h review explicitly scored

Domain	PLAB 2	UKMLA CPSA
Safeguarding	FGM · domestic abuse · child protection	Same · Modern slavery and trafficking more likely
Mental health	MSE · capacity · risk assessment	Same · Trauma-informed care language expected
Documentation	Verbal: "I would document..."	Same verbal approach · may be asked to write brief note
Pass standard	UK Foundation Programme readiness	Same standard
Covered by this series?	✓ Yes — fully	✓ Yes — fully

EDI Note for UKMLA Candidates:
The UKMLA explicitly scores equity, diversity, and inclusion behaviours. In practice this means: avoid assumptions based on gender, ethnicity, religion, or background · use inclusive language · acknowledge cultural factors in health beliefs · ask "What matters to you?" not just "What is the problem?"
All of these behaviours are already embedded in the ICE framework and empathy scripts throughout this series. No additional preparation needed.

Final Mantra

Every fail in every vignette was a behaviour, not a knowledge gap. Know the patterns. Recognise them in yourself. Fix them before the exam.
Safety domain = binary. One breach = fail regardless of everything else. All other domains = recoverable.
ICE alone is worth 2–4 marks per station. Safety-net is worth 1–2. Allergy check is 2 free marks. These are the easiest marks in the exam — and the most commonly dropped.
PLAB 2 and UKMLA: same system, same standards, same this series.

Safety = auto fail all other domains recover	**ICE = 4 marks** most commonly dropped	**Allergy check = free** 2 marks in 5 seconds	**Silence = no marks** verbalise everything	**MTX daily = fail** once weekly always
10 vignettes all behaviour not knowledge	**Conditional apology fails** I'm sorry you feel that way	**Promised secrecy fails** safeguarding = share	**PLAB2 = UKMLA** same system same series	**Reset between stations** carry nothing forward

Appendix 3I · Instant-Fail Behaviours Quick Reminder

Condensed reference · Full version in Volume 1 (App 1B)

True Failure Causes: Safety breach · Consent violation · Suicide mismanagement · Safeguarding failure · Major prescribing error · Professionalism lapse

#	Category	Key Instant-Fail Behaviours
1	Consent & Capacity	No consent · No chaperone (intimate exam) · Continue after refusal · Ignore capacity issues
2	Clinical Danger	Send high-risk chest pain home · Miss cauda equina · No ABCDE in collapse · No O_2 in hypoxia
3	Prescribing	Prescribe despite allergy · 10× dose error · No allergy check · Contraindicated in pregnancy
4	Safeguarding	Ignore child protection · Ignore abuse disclosure · Promise secrecy
5	Suicide & MH	No suicide screen when indicated · Miss intent/plan · Discharge high-risk without safety plan
6	Ethics	Breach confidentiality · Lie to patient · Falsify documentation
7	Bad News	No warning shot · Never says "cancer" clearly · Continue while patient is crying

SAFE Rule: Safety first · Ask ICE + assess risk · Flag emergencies · Explain clearly + safety-net

Subtle Fatal Combinations (Tier 2):

Poor empathy + unsafe discharge · No ICE + imposed plan · No suicide screen + false reassurance

Appendix 3J · Station Micro-Summary Quick Reminder

Condensed reference · Full version in Volume 1 (App 1D)

Top 5 Must-Say Phrases:
ICE: "What do you think? Any worries? What were you hoping for?"
Safety-Net: "Return if symptoms worsen, new symptoms appear, or you're worried."
Escalate: "I would discuss this with my senior."
Empathy: "That sounds really difficult."
SDM: "Some prefer X, others Y — what are your thoughts?"

H	HISTORY	Hello · ICE · Set agenda · Take history (SOCRATES) · Other background · Reflect · Your safety-net
S	SAFE PLAN	Summarise safety · Assess · Formulate 5Ps · Explain SDM · Liaise/escalate · Arrange follow-up · Never forget safety-net
B	BREAKDOWN	Begin permission · Results · Explain simply · Assess understanding · Keep ICE · Discuss options · Offer written info · Wonder about questions · Next steps
B	BRIDGE	Build rapport · Recognise emotion · ICE deep dive · Don't argue, bridge · Give info gently · Explore options collaboratively

2-Minute Flow: Before: hygiene + observe · First 30s: introduce + ICE · Middle: signpost + template + empathy + verbalise · End: SDM + safety-net + close + document
Emergency Override: Patient unstable → STOP. Switch to ABCDE. Call for help. Resume only when safe.

APPENDIX S · MASTER MNEMONIC INDEX

All mnemonics alphabetically · Quick lookup for last-minute revision

AMaC · PLAB 2 Master Series · Volume 3

How to use: Find any mnemonic alphabetically. The Volume column shows which volume contains it. The Expansion gives enough of the trigger phrase to reconstruct the full framework from memory.

Volume 1 = Foundations · Volume 2 = Clinical Medicine · Volume 3 = Procedures & Mock

Mnemonic	Vol	Expansion · Key phrase	Location
ABCDE	V1	Airway · Breathing · Circulation · Disability · Exposure	*Emergency framework — every acute station*
AEIOU-TIPS	V1	Alcohol · Epilepsy · Insulin · Uraemia · Overdose · Trauma · Infection · Psychiatric · Stroke (causes of reduced consciousness)	*Ch 17*
BRIDGE	V1	Brief · Rapport · Involve · Don't argue · Give options · Explore (difficult conversations)	*App 1D*
BREAKDOWN	V1	Brief · Red flags · Explain · Assess · Knowledgecheck · Down-chunk · Options · Wait · Next steps (explanation stations)	*App 1D*
BUFALO	V1	Blood cultures · Urine output · Fluids · Antibiotics · Lactate · Oxygen (Sepsis-6)	*Ch 13*
HISTORY	V1	History template mnemonic (history stations)	*App 1D*
ICE	V1	Ideas · Concerns · Expectations	*Ch 1 — every station*
MR-SOPA	V1	Mask · Reposition · Suction · Open mouth · Pressure increase · Airway alternative (neonatal PPV)	*Ch 10*
NURSE	V1	Name emotion · Understand · Respect · Support · Explore (empathy framework)	*Ch 2*
SAFE-CALL	V1	Safety identity · Allergy · Formulate history · Escalate if needed · Call back plan · Link to urgent care (remote consultation)	*Ch 7*
SAFE-DOC	V1	Safety · Allergy · Facts · Evidence · Date/time · Other clinicians · Consequences (documentation)	*Ch 5*
SAFE-PLAN	V1	Safe management plan template (management stations)	*App 1D*
SBAR	V1	Situation · Background · Assessment · Recommendation	*Ch 3 — every handover*
SPIKES	V1	Setting · Perception · Invitation · Knowledge · Empathy · Strategy (breaking bad news)	*Ch 2*

Mnemonic	Vol	Expansion · Key phrase	Location
URWC	**V1**	Understand · Retain · Weigh up · Communicate (capacity assessment)	*Ch 2*
6-PACK	**V2**	Prioritise targets · Individualise · Assess complications · Cardiovascular risk · Knowledge/safety · Tailor care (diabetes annual review)	*Ch 30*
AIRWAY-FIRST	**V2**	Assess from doorway · Immediate senior call · No distressing interventions · Upright position · When to intubate (upper airway emergency)	*Ch 28*
BABY-CHECK	**V2**	Booking tests · Anomaly scan · Bloods · Yell for help if unwell · Check BP/urine · History · Engage safeguarding · Close safety-net · Keys for referral (antenatal)	*Ch 33*
CORD	**V2**	Cancer history · Onset back pain · Radicular pain · Disability: leg weakness+sensory+bladder (cord compression)	*Ch 39*
CUP-FIRST	**V2**	Cu-IUD first · UPA second · LNG third (emergency contraception hierarchy)	*Ch 32*
EYE-TIME	**V2**	Eye emergency framework for acute vision loss — identify type first	*Ch 27*
FRAILY	**V2**	Falls · Review medications · Assessment cognition (4AT) · Integration carer · Levels of risk (safeguarding) · Your baseline (ADLs)	*Ch 37*
HELPERR	**V2**	Help call · Episiotomy · Legs McRoberts · Pressure suprapubic · Enter rotation · Remove arm · Roll (shoulder dystocia)	*Ch 43*
PINCH-ME	**V2**	Pain · Infection · Nutrition · Constipation · Hydration · Medication · Environment (delirium causes)	*Ch 37*
SADMAN	**V2**	SGLT2i · ACEi/ARBs · Diuretics · Metformin · Monitor glucose · NSAIDs (sick-day rules — stop these)	*Ch 30/35*
SAD-C	**V2**	Septic arthritis · Angioedema · Diphtheria · Croup / Bacterial tracheitis (stridor differential)	*Ch 28*
SAFER-SEX	**V2**	Sexual history framework for contraception/STI stations	*Ch 32*
SHARP	**V2**	Shoulder tip pain · Hypotension · Adrenaline-like signs · Rigid abdomen · Peritonism (ectopic rupture)	*Ch 42*
SICK-RASH	**V2**	Septicaemia · Immune/HSP · Cellulitis · Kawasaki · Rash+fever rule · All = emergency until proven (paediatric rash)	*Ch 47*
TARGET	**V2**	Treatment burden · Age · Risk of hypoglycaemia · Goals · Existing complications · Time to benefit (HbA1c individualisation)	*Ch 30*

Mnemonic	Vol	Expansion · Key phrase	Location
TWIST	V2	Testicular swelling · Wall thickening · Ischaemia · Solid mass · Tenderness (testicular torsion score)	*Ch 29*
ABDOMEN	V3	Appearance · Bowel sounds · Dullness · Organomegaly · Masses · End tests · Negatives (abdominal examination)	*Ch 59*
ASEPTIC	V3	Appearance · Speech · Emotion · Perception · Thought · Insight · Cognition (MSE)	*Ch 62*
BAD	V3	Big problems first: pH <7.2 · Alarmingly high CO_2 · Dangerously low HCO_3 (ABG first-look scan)	*Ch 70*
CANNULA	V3	Cannulation procedure mnemonic	*Ch 63*
CLEAN-GO	V3	Catheterisation procedure — male (Clean · Lube · Erect · Advance · No force · Go/CUFI)	*Ch 64*
CLEAN-SEE	V3	Catheterisation procedure — female (Clean · Locate · Enter · Advance · No force · See/CUFI)	*Ch 64*
CONSENT	V3	Capacity · Open questions · No pressure · Sufficient info · Explicit yes · Note · Time (consent process)	*Ch 57*
CUFI	V3	Check urine freely flowing · Urine confirmed in bladder · Fill balloon slowly · Inflate watching for pain	*Ch 64*
EXAMINE	V3	Explicit consent · eXplain · Ask comfort · Minimal exposure · Involve chaperone · Never silent · End with summary	*Ch 57*
IOAPM	V3	Insulin · Opioids · Anticoagulants · Potassium IV · Methotrexate (highest-risk injectable drugs)	*Ch 67*
IPPA-C	V3	Inspection · Palpation · Percussion · Auscultation · Complete special tests (respiratory examination)	*Ch 58*
KILL	V3	K+ changes · Ischaemia · Lethal rhythms (VT/VF/Torsades) · Low rate/heart block (ECG 5-sec danger scan)	*Ch 70*
LA-TIP	V3	Local anaesthetic safety rule	*Ch 65*
ORIP	V3	Once daily · Regular · IV · PRN (prescribing sections)	*Ch 67*
PALPATE	V3	Position · Ask pain · Light palpation · Palpate deep · Assess organs · Tenderness · Examine orifices	*Ch 59*
PERFECT	V3	Position · Exposure · Rate/rhythm · Feel (apex) · Edge (borders) · Characterise murmur · Thrills/heaves (CVS examination)	*Ch 58*

Mnemonic	Vol	Expansion · Key phrase	Location
PINK	V3	Pressing emergency → PCC+VitK · Intermediate → VitK alone · Nil urgency → hold warfarin (warfarin reversal)	Ch 68
PREPARE	V3	Permission · Reason · Explain · Position · Ask comfort · Reassure · End with summary (examination opener)	Ch 57
RAMP	V3	Renal (eGFR <30) · Allergy (contrast) · Metformin (withhold 48h) · Pregnancy (avoid if possible) — pre-contrast checklist	Ch 71
RIPE	V3	Rotation · Inspiration (≥6 ribs) · Projection (clavicle/spine) · Exposure (lung bases visible) — CXR quality check	Ch 71
ROME	V3	Respiratory = Opposite direction to pH · Metabolic = Equal/same direction (acid-base disorder rule)	Ch 70
RRAIS	V3	Rate · Rhythm · Axis · Intervals · ST/T changes (ECG systematic approach)	Ch 70
SAFE-TIE	V3	Suturing pre-procedure safety framework	Ch 65
SCAN-60	V3	K+≥6 · Glucose<3 · Lactate>4 · Hb<70 · eGFR<30 · Na+<120 or >155 (blood test danger thresholds)	Ch 72
WISE	V3	Watch level · Inspect drain · Swinging · Examine bubbling (chest drain monitoring)	Ch 66
WILM-NOSABDG	V3	Warfarin · Insulin · Lithium · MTX · NSAIDs · Opioids · Steroids · ACEi · Beta-blockers · Diuretics · Gentamicin (high-risk drugs)	Ch 68

MASTER GLOSSARY · ABBREVIATIONS

Abbrev	Meaning	Abbrev	Meaning
ACL	Anterior Cruciate Ligament	**MHA**	Mental Health Act
ACS	Acute Coronary Syndrome	**MMR**	Measles, Mumps & Rubella
AKI	Acute Kidney Injury	**MRC**	Medical Research Council scale
AMT-10	Abbreviated Mental Test (10-point)	**MSE**	Mental State Examination
BMV	Bag-Mask Ventilation	**MTP**	Metatarsophalangeal joint
BNF	British National Formulary	**MTX**	Methotrexate
BTS	British Thoracic Society	**NBM**	Nil By Mouth
CAP	Community-Acquired Pneumonia	**NEWS2**	National Early Warning Score 2
CHB	Complete Heart Block	**NIV**	Non-Invasive Ventilation
CIWA	Clinical Institute Withdrawal Assessment	**NKDA**	No Known Drug Allergies
CKD	Chronic Kidney Disease	**NPA**	Nasopharyngeal Airway
CN	Cranial Nerve	**NSAID**	Non-Steroidal Anti-Inflammatory Drug
COPD	Chronic Obstructive Pulmonary Disease	**NSTEMI**	Non-ST-Elevation Myocardial Infarction
CPAP	Continuous Positive Airway Pressure	**OPA**	Oropharyngeal Airway
CPSA	Clinical & Procedural Skills Assessment	**PCC**	Prothrombin Complex Concentrate
CTG	Cardiotocography	**PCI**	Percutaneous Coronary Intervention
CURB-65	CURB-65 pneumonia severity score	**PE**	Pulmonary Embolism
DKA	Diabetic Ketoacidosis	**PLAB**	Professional & Linguistic Assessments Board
DNACPR	Do Not Attempt Cardiopulmonary Resuscitation	**PPH**	Postpartum Haemorrhage
DVLA	Driver & Vehicle Licensing Agency	**PPI**	Proton Pump Inhibitor
DVT	Deep Vein Thrombosis	**RCUK**	Resuscitation Council UK
EBL	Estimated Blood Loss	**RUQ**	Right Upper Quadrant
EOM	Extraocular Movements	**RV**	Right Ventricle
FGM	Female Genital Mutilation	**SAH**	Subarachnoid Haemorrhage

FM	Fetal Movements	**SBP**	Systolic Blood Pressure
GDM	Gestational Diabetes Mellitus	**STEMI**	ST-Elevation Myocardial Infarction
GTN	Glyceryl Trinitrate	**SVC**	Superior Vena Cava
HCM	Hypertrophic Cardiomyopathy	**SVT**	Supraventricular Tachycardia
HF	Heart Failure	**TMJ**	Temporomandibular Joint
ICH	Intracranial Haemorrhage	**TTO**	To-Take-Out (discharge) medication
ICP	Intracranial Pressure	**UKMLA**	UK Medical Licensing Assessment
IUD	Intrauterine Device	**UMN**	Upper Motor Neurone
IUGR	Intrauterine Growth Restriction	**UPA**	Ulipristal Acetate
JVP	Jugular Venous Pressure	**URTI**	Upper Respiratory Tract Infection
LBBB	Left Bundle Branch Block	**USS**	Ultrasound Scan
LMN	Lower Motor Neurone	**VF**	Ventricular Fibrillation
LNG	Levonorgestrel	**VR**	Vocal Resonance
LP	Lumbar Puncture	**VRIII**	Variable Rate Intravenous Insulin Infusion
MCL	Mid-Clavicular Line / Medial Collateral Ligament	**VT**	Ventricular Tachycardia
MCP	Metacarpophalangeal joint	**WOB**	Work of Breathing
MDT	Multidisciplinary Team		

www.ingramcontent.com/pod-product-compliance
Lightning Source LLC
LaVergne TN
LVHW010722061126
851857LV00014B/1304